Anti-vaxxers

Anti-vaxxers

How to Challenge a Misinformed Movement

Jonathan M. Berman

The MIT Press
Cambridge, Massachusetts
London, England

This book was set in Stone Serif and Stone Sans by Westchester Publishing Services. Printed and bound in the United States of America.

Library of Congress Cataloging-in-Publication Data

Names: Berman, Jonathan M., author.
Title: Anti-vaxxers : how to challenge a misinformed movement / Jonathan M. Berman.
Description: Cambridge, Massachusetts : The MIT Press, [2020] | Includes bibliographical references and index.
Identifiers: LCCN 2019057058 | ISBN 9780262539326 (paperback)
Subjects: MESH: Anti-Vaccination Movement | Vaccination Refusal | Sociological Factors | Vaccination—psychology | Treatment Outcome | United States
Classification: LCC RA638 | NLM WA 115 | DDC 614.4/7—dc23
LC record available at https://lccn.loc.gov/2019057058

10 9 8 7 6 5 4 3 2 1

Contents

Preface

Most of this book was written in 2018 and 2019, before the onset of the global COVID-19 pandemic that rages as I write this preface. In January 2020 I started watching news of the pandemic closely, and I started examining how people on the internet reacted to the news. A Reddit user posted an analysis that they claimed showed that the Chinese government was lying because the number of new (at the time called 2019-nCoV) cases fit better to a quadratic regression than exponential. I started examining the published epidemiological numbers on the epidemic, and because I'm not an epidemiologist, I didn't believe that I had run the analysis correctly.

The model I ran predicted that in the United States, if COVID-19 became common, as many as 4 million people would die. It seemed an impossibly high number. Surely I had misunderstood a variable. In February 2020, a medical student who was doing a fellowship in a congressional office asked me about the outbreak in China, and I showed her my analysis. I included a figure with the effects of reductions in potentially infectious interactions being reduced in increments by 0 percent, 20 percent, 40 percent, 60 percent, and so on. The figure showed that if interactions were reduced by 40 percent, it would buy scientists time to study the new disease, and give physicians time to treat it. I warned her that the state I live in has a limited number of hospital beds. I did not anticipate a shortage of ventilators, masks, or toilet paper. Later, someone presented a much clearer figure that showed the same idea. If we practiced "social distancing," by isolating ourselves and minimizing our interactions with other people, we could slow the spread of the disease.

As the nature of COVID-19 became clear, a global pandemic was declared, and individual businesses, universities, cities and states started to implement shutdowns; but politicians were slow to respond. Some downplayed it, by comparing it to seasonal flu, which is widespread and kills tens of thousands every year, but which the current healthcare system can mostly handle. Some, watching the stock market lose value, floated the idea that the death of the elderly was an acceptable sacrifice to ward off an economic recession. Worldwide, there have been reports of individuals ignoring the warnings of scientists and public health offices, going about their daily lives as if nothing unusual were going on.

While anti-vaccine activists won't be relevant to the current crisis until a vaccine is developed, tested, and brought to market, the behavior of people who have ignored lockdowns or left quarantine to attend parties shares some similarities. In South Korea, a woman refused testing, despite showing symptoms and infected dozens of others by continuing to attend church. In Kentucky, young people defied state guidance to stay home and threw a "coronavirus party" where a partygoer infected at least one other. In Florida, college students gathered at beaches to celebrate spring break. Said one: "If I get corona, I get corona. At the end of the day, I'm not going to let it stop me." Later some students who had gathered in Florida tested positive for SARS-COV-2 (the virus that causes COVID-19). Large churches have continued to hold services with thousands of attendees, despite state orders. Liberty University reopened amid the crisis. US Senator Rand Paul was tested, and continued to gather with other lawmakers and use the senate gym for several days before his results returned positive and he began self-isolating. Some large churches have continued to hold services with thousands of attendees.

We are early in the pandemic, and it's likely that these "anti-social-distancers" will be studied in depth in the coming years. However, some traits seem to stand out: a lack of trust in medical authorities, a misunderstanding of the scale of human suffering that infectious disease can impart, ignorance of science, and a tendency to make comparisons between SARS-COV-2 and seasonal flu.

The toll that flu takes each year is indeed steep. According to CDC estimates, each year tens of thousands of Americans die due to influenza and its complications. But influenza differs from SARS-COV-2 in some important ways. First, each year a vaccine is developed which allows for some protection against influenza. Influenza also appears to be less contagious than SARS-COV-2. Someone with influenza infects about 1.3 other people on average over the course of their infection. It currently appears that someone with SARS-COV-2 infects about twice that many. A greater percentage of people suffering from COVID-19 (up to 20 percent) require hospitalization, and a greater percentage of those who require hospitalization die. New (as of late March 2020) evidence suggests that a large portion of those who test positive for SARS-COV-2 are totally asymptomatic and capable of infecting others without realizing it. Together these features make SARS-COV-2 significantly more dangerous than seasonal influenza, because it can spread rapidly and overwhelm hospital systems, which are typically built with little overload capacity. Already, Italy has suffered greatly under shortages of personal protective equipment such as masks, as well as equipment such as ventilators, and similar shortages are anticipated in New York and other areas of the United States.

The apparently high proportion of asymptomatic carriers of SARS-CoV-2 seems to encourage anti-social-distancers. Owing to an early shortage of testing materials, tests were available only to those meeting very specific conditions. However, it is becoming clear that a high fraction of those who have been infected show no symptoms at all. Many who should have been quarantined have been free to travel without realizing that they were spreading disease, including some who went out of their way to travel and continue to meet up with others.

Complicating this in the United States has been a partisan political response to the pandemic. So far large, densely populated cities have been the hardest hit, and less-populated rural areas have not yet seen infection rates as high. The urban rural divide underlies much of the political disagreement in the United States, and this has been reflected in polling that shows that the degree of concern people have about COVID-19 is heavily dependent on their political leaning. Some partisan news sources initially downplayed the severity of COVID-19, and took cues from politicians who seemed to want to reopen businesses that had been closed due to social-distancing regardless of the cost in human lives. Similar partisan responses have occurred in other countries. In Brazil, President Jair Bolsonaro has publicly called for reopening businesses and has continued to go out in public denying the severity of COVID-19 and attempting to undermine regional government's efforts to shut down. Bolsonaro was quoted as saying, "Some will die. I'm sorry. That's life."

One thing is certain: life has changed for millions of people around the world in this crisis. It has forced many who grew up in an era and location where infectious disease was not confronted or dealt with on a daily basis to confront the dreadful facts of a pandemic. Personally, I have shut down my lab, and may travel to the state capital in a few days to volunteer in the public health lab, testing samples. The nature of such fast-moving events means that much of this note will be outdated by the time you read this. However, I hope that this book about anti-vaccine activists gives some insight into anti-social distancers as well.

Introduction

The broad class of treatments collectively referred to as vaccines has been instrumental in eliminating some diseases, severely reducing the incidence of others, and helping to reduce the overall incidence of infectious disease as a cause of death. Vaccines have significantly reduced the burden of human suffering. Their story is one of the great tales of human progress and our ability to develop tools and knowledge that allow us to improve our quality of life. Nevertheless, some people oppose vaccination vehemently.

Although many attribute the modern anti-vaccine movement to Andrew Wakefield, and his 1998 paper purporting to link the measles, mumps, and rubella vaccine to the development of a kind of late-onset autism, opposition to vaccination is not new. Since the first smallpox vaccine was invented at the turn of the nineteenth century, there has been opposition to vaccination.[1] In the case of the first vaccination, this opposition may have been justified because an uneducated farmer used a darning needle to acquire pus from an infected cow's udders and then scratch his family members. These historic anti-vaccine movements have much to teach us about the modern anti-vaccine movement.

Wakefield's paper followed decades of anti-vaccine rhetoric in the nineteenth and twentieth centuries. This rhetoric was driven by changing views on bodily autonomy, the role of the state in medical care, fears held over from the rollout of the first polio vaccines, and an earlier scare surrounding the diphtheria, tetanus, and pertussis vaccine that started in 1974. The vaccine scare of the 1970s and 1980s carried through to the 1990s, forcing several vaccine manufacturers out of business. Although Wakefield's paper was one of many proximate causes of the modern anti-vaccination movement, it received widespread press attention—far more than did subsequent papers that did not support its conclusions.[2] We will look at questions about the interface between news media and science, as well as at questions about how fake news spreads faster than real news.

Over the last two and a quarter centuries, this opposition has been driven by several motivators: fear of adverse side effects, objection to government intrusion in the body, conspiracy theories about "Big Pharma," the financial motivation of those selling "alternative" treatments and of lawyers seeking to sue drug companies, fear of Western or colonial intrusion into communities, rejection of the idea that anyone but a child's own parents might know what's best for them, and a sense of community and identity built around parenting choices.

This opposition has caused real harm over time, including deaths from outbreaks of smallpox, measles, and polio; bankruptcy of vaccine manufacturers leading to shortages; and personal heartbreak as divisions sown by anti-vaccine activists have damaged family relationships and friendships.

Despite these setbacks, overall vaccination rates are high worldwide, and anti-vaccine activism is still a niche pursuit. However, small enclaves exist where anti-vaccine rhetoric has been effective, leading to clusters of unvaccinated children. These clusters put at risk those who for a variety of medical reasons may not be able to vaccinate, and have led to outbreaks of chickenpox and measles.

Three broad strategies have been used to sway people from anti-vaccine beliefs. I refer to these as reactive, information-deficit, and community-based strategies. A reactive strategy of engaging directly with anti-vaccine advocates on the internet and mocking them or arguing with them is the least effective. Not only are vocal online anti-vaccine advocates not representative of the average person with vaccine doubts, but this strategy can backfire, resulting in more entrenched views and damaged family relationships.

When anti-vaccine activists cite scientific articles or use the language of evidence, typically they are aiming to justify beliefs that are held for non-evidence-based reasons. Addressing an argument without addressing the underlying emotional reasons for a belief is unlikely to be effective. When opposition to vaccination becomes attached to a person's identity and values, contradictory information can feel like an attack on that identity and those values.

Information-deficit strategies approach vaccination by making factual information about vaccination available to the public through, for example, websites, internet resources, and fact sheets. While presenting information resources to the public has been successful in increasing the intent to vaccinate, these strategies require those with questions to seek out such resources in the first place and then to know which of them are trustworthy. These strategies are not likely to be effective for entrenched anti-vaccine activists but can be effective for those with questions or doubts.

Community-based strategies, which I believe to be most effective, are strategies based on showing those with doubts that others in their community are vaccinating their children; that their peers in their mosque, synagogue, church, or temple who are also good parents have vaccinated their children; and that vaccination is an expectation of any good parent. Community-based strategies have been used in the wake of measles outbreaks exacerbated by anti-vaccine activism and resulted in significant increases in vaccine uptake. These strategies take into consideration the self-identity and values of those who are being targeted by anti-vaccine rhetoric.

This book presents information that fits with all three strategies. It refutes many specific claims made by anti-vaccine activists. Those seeking more details on these claims can look to additional resources, such as Paul Offit's books or Seth Mnookin's *The Panic Virus*. I have endeavored to balance not providing an additional platform to anti-vaccine activists with addressing some of their most prominent and visible claims.

There is an inherent tension in seeking to understand a movement while simultaneously refuting its claims. In this case, these goals are not truly at odds. There is no single organized anti-vaccine movement. There are many individuals who have been influenced by a specific set of beliefs. An important part of understanding those beliefs is understanding if they are true.

I doubt that a reader approaching this book with entrenched anti-vaccine views is likely to have her or his mind changed. However, many have encountered conflicting information about vaccines or heard negative information from friends and relatives but don't necessarily know enough about the topic to form a strong opinion either way. Others know about the importance of vaccination but would benefit from a deeper discussion of the history of the anti-vaccine movement when having an informed discussion about it.

We will explore the motivations of anti-vaccine advocates, including those with strong financial incentives, such as those selling "alternative" treatments; otherwise good, well-intended parents who have gotten bad information; and internet activists with myriad techniques and means of spreading misinformation. We will explore some of the psychological effects that make these techniques effective in spreading information and the means by which those with good information can work toward meaningful change in the laws regarding nonmedical exemptions.

As we discuss religious exemptions, it will become clear that few religions actually specify an opposition to vaccination in their official teachings. Providing these exemptions harms those who have legitimate medical reasons for being unable to receive vaccines, such as donor organ recipients, those with compromised immune systems, and the extremely young and extremely old.

We will also discuss those harmed indirectly by the anti-vaccine movement, not just those who become sick but also disability advocates, a daughter estranged from her own mother because of a rift opened by her mother's anti-vaccine sentiment, and activists who have received death threats for working on public health initiatives. Determining whether or not to receive vaccinations involves a set of decisions, each of which carries moral weight. They are decisions with the power to create or ease suffering. So this book also touches very lightly on moral philosophy.

In this book I have two goals. The first is to provide a more complete picture of the anti-vaccine movement, from its inception in the nineteenth century to present-day social-media wars. This goal is undertaken with the understanding that there is a complex balance of risks that we must face when making decisions about our own and others' health, and which decision is correct can be murky and clouded with misinformation. I hope that this book brings the reader a deeper understanding of the anti-vaccine movement.

The second goal is to provide a counterpoint to some of the misinformation to which the reader may already have been exposed. If you are on the fence and looking for more information, then I hope this book will serve as a good resource. If you are opposed to vaccination, then I hope you will approach this book with an open mind.

1   Is There Even a Problem?

Is the anti-vaccination movement even significant enough to pose a widespread threat to public health? To answer that question, we must look at actual immunization rates. If immunization rates were universally meeting targets and outbreaks of preventable disease were not occurring, then anti-vaccine activists would be unworthy of notice or response.

As of 2016 vaccine coverage in the United States exceeded targets for vaccination with diphtheria, tetanus, and pertussis (DTaP); poliovirus; measles, mumps, and rubella (MMR); haemophilus influenzae B (Hib); hepatitis B (HepB); varicella; pneumococcal conjugate (PCV); hepatitis A (HepA); and rotavirus.[1] Coverage did not statistically change from 2012 to 2016. For most of these vaccines, coverage was above targets of 90 percent, but for vaccines that required boosters during the second year of life, coverage was somewhat lower. The best predictors of vaccine coverage were not membership in anti-vaccine groups but access to medical care as determined by private insurance coverage, race, and socioeconomic status.

In the United States, overall rates of people seeking exemptions based on philosophical beliefs are low, and religious objections are even lower. From 2011 to 2012, exemption rates for the MMR vaccine were less than or equal to 2 percent.[2] Rates in Europe are similar. Although more Europeans express skepticism about vaccination, this has not in most cases translated into action significant enough to cause outbreaks of disease. In France, as of 2016, 41 percent of respondents disagreed or strongly disagreed with the statement "Overall I think vaccines are safe,"[3] yet 96 percent of children were vaccinated against diphtheria, tetanus, and pertussis, and 89 percent of children were vaccinated against measles.[4] These numbers are lower than would be ideal but are not as bad as suggested by the level of vaccine doubt. The difference between vaccine doubt and vaccination rate is a gap between intent and action.

This disparity between belief and behavior has been termed the intention-behavior gap,[5] or the value-action gap. Many of us experience such gaps in our daily lives. Most smokers know that smoking is bad for them but smoke anyway. We know that driving above the speed limit is dangerous, but most drivers occasionally exceed speed limits. It isn't that smokers don't value their health but that various other factors enter into each decision to smoke. Likewise there are many factors that affect the likelihood of an individual choosing to vaccinate. While the measles-vaccination rate in France should be higher, and the French government is working to improve vaccine coverage, the factors affecting parents' decisions to vaccinate include more than doubts alone.

Those vaccines that have faced difficulty achieving high coverage rates are often tied to other controversies of morality or identity. Gardasil—a vaccine against some strains of the human papillomavirus, HPV, that causes almost all cervical and anal cancers, as well as the majority of vaginal cancers and cancers of the tonsils, soft palate, and base of the tongue[6]—became very controversial after it was approved. Several largely Christian religious groups opposed adding Gardasil to routine vaccination schedules on the basis that they believed it would lead young women to having premarital sex,[7] which they opposed. Opposition to the HPV vaccine is probably better explained by the moral and cultural identity of those opposing it than by opposition to vaccination as a whole.

The way that Gardasil was introduced by Merck & Co. Inc. may have played a role in this controversy,[8] as well as in reporting in the media that did not properly place the data and the opposition to the vaccine in context.[9] Merck enacted a lobbying campaign in state legislatures to make Gardasil mandatory for young girls. The campaign produced a very negative public reaction.[10] By comparison, the HepB vaccine, which similarly treats a sexually transmitted infection that can cause cancers, was introduced without much controversy and added to the routine childhood immunization schedule in the 1990s. The way that vaccines are introduced—as well as the cultural competency of those introducing them—to communities plays a very important role in preventing vaccine hesitancy.

Despite the overall high vaccination rates in the United States, there are enclaves where anti-vaccine rhetoric has taken root, and decreases in immunization rates have occurred, leading to outbreaks in some cases. As early as 2010, anti-vaccine activists were speaking to the Somali-American community in Minnesota.[11] In April through August 2017, there was a measles outbreak in Minnesota, the largest in thirty years, with seventy-nine cases, most of them Somali-American children. This outbreak had the potential to be far worse because measles-vaccination rates, while overall high, were much lower in some groups, such as private schools, where the vaccination coverage averaged only 83 percent.[12] In a remarkable collaboration, public health officials worked with

Somali-American imams to conduct a vaccination campaign.[13] Between April and July 2017, more than triple the normal number of vaccinations occurred in Minnesota clinics, and after the end of the outbreak, vaccination rates remained higher than before the outbreak.[14] These results suggest that culturally literate approaches to communities where vaccination has declined can be effective in fighting outbreaks. Reports at the time showed people handing out fliers to spread anti-vaccine conspiracy theories in the Somali-American community, although anti-vaccine groups campaigning in the area denied this activity.

In another example, in 2014 through 2015, a measles outbreak occurred in California that spread to over one hundred children, 45 percent of whom were unvaccinated.[15] In the news media, this became known as the Disneyland outbreak. In California, vaccination rates had dropped from above 95 percent to about 92 percent in the prior decade, an effect attributed to anti-vaccine activism. Following the outbreak, several public health measures were taken.[16] A law, SB-277, made it more difficult to obtain nonmedical vaccine exemptions for children entering public school, and the University of California system refused to accept unvaccinated freshmen. As a result, childhood vaccination rates have risen to above pre-2004 levels. However, some counties still lag behind others in vaccination rates because there is still a cohort of children who were never vaccinated under the previous, rather lax criteria.

In 2019 an outbreak spread to over a thousand cases, a number much higher than the number of cases in the United States in any previous year since measles was declared eliminated in the country in 2000.[17] The outbreak began in an Orthodox Jewish community in New York when an unvaccinated child returned from Israel carrying the virus. In Washington State, where Clark County saw seventy-three cases of measles, the state government passed House Bill 1638, which eliminated personal- and philosophical-belief vaccine exemptions in the state but still allowed religious exemptions.[18] We will see in a later chapter that religious exemptions are rarely based on the teachings of any religion and often invite parents to lie. In Rockland County, New York, a law banning unvaccinated minors from public spaces was passed[19]; however, this ban was placed on hold.[20] As part of the outbreak, a US cruise ship, operated by the Church of Scientology, was quarantined due to measles risk[21] but later cleared.

Despite the relatively high vaccination rates in almost all countries with vaccine doubt, Ukraine stands as an outlier, with both high vaccine doubt and a drop in vaccination rates for polio, measles, mumps, and rubella to around 50 percent. This drop preceded a measles outbreak.[22] In Ukraine, vaccination is required prior to school attendance. However, it was often easier to obtain a fake certificate than to obtain a vaccination due to hospitals running low on free vaccines. This forced parents to face paying high costs at pharmacies. More than half of the more than forty thousand cases of measles in Europe in 2018 were in Ukraine.[23] The decline in Ukrainian MMR-vaccination rates from 95 percent in 2008 to 31 percent in 2016 was astonishing, and even the current 85 percent rate is below that required to prevent transmission in the population. This drop in vaccination rates may have been caused in part by Russia-backed Twitter accounts that sought to spread misinformation about vaccines[24] and to create false equivalency between pro- and anti-vaccine arguments.

The biggest rate-limiting factor to vaccination is the availability of vaccines. Where availability is high, even those with doubts tend to become vaccinated or have their children vaccinated. Where availability is impeded by cost or other impediments,

Anti-vaccine activists have been successful in limited ways by establishing doubt within isolated communities. In the United States, when rates have dropped low enough in enclaves that an outbreak occurs, historically, the reaction has been swift, culturally competent, and very effective in recovering vaccination rates. In absolute numbers, the number of children who have died because of these outbreaks in the United States is low.

These data are heartening because they show that the overall impact of the anti-vaccine movement has been low. However, if you are a parent or relative of a child who does become infected with a vaccine-preventable illness, your child is still sick. If you are a parent whose children attend school, you will have an interest in knowing that your community has high vaccination rates. If you are the parent of an immunocompromised child who is unable to be vaccinated, membership in a community where immunization rates are high is an important step in protecting your child's life. Oscillations between minor outbreaks and adequate vaccination rates is less desirable than eliminating those diseases or maintaining a high steady state of vaccination.

Public health efforts to eliminate diseases have so far eliminated only two worldwide, smallpox and rinderpest. The goal of eliminating polio by 2015 has been missed, and it seems unlikely to be eliminated by 2020, although the cases of wild polio have decreased to the low double digits, and elimination still appears to be an achievable near-term goal.

All politics is local.
—attributed to Tip O'Neill

Because the risks of the anti-vaccine movement take place at the level of local communities, schools, preschools, churches,

2   Understanding Vaccines

We first need to understand what vaccines are, a little bit about how they work, and the circumstances when we *should* vaccinate. This book sometimes treats vaccination as a single action and vaccines as a single entity. Of course, this is not fully accurate. There is more than one kind of vaccine, and vaccines may be targeted against infectious diseases caused by bacteria, viruses, fungi, or animal parasites, or they may be targeted against cancer. Vaccines may be composed of many different substances and may be administered under very different circumstances. However, because the anti-vaccine movement often discusses vaccination as a single action, our discussion of vaccination will sometimes adopt this language so that we can discuss and address the movement's claims.

A vaccine is an agent that creates immunity against a disease-causing agent (*pathogen*) without causing the disease itself. Immunity is the collection of defenses against disease-causing organisms and materials, as well as cancer cells, that allows us to maintain protection against outside invasion. This system is both remarkable, in the efficiency with which it protects us, and imperfect.

Immunity begins with passive physical and chemical barriers that insulate our internal environment from the external. For example, the skin forms a continuous barrier that is capable of preventing the majority of microorganisms from entering our bodies. Pathogens on the surface of the skin can dry out and can be attacked by the acidity of human skin. An invading pathogen must also compete with the natural flora that already populates human skin. A classic experiment in introductory microbiology classes for undergraduates involves swabbing the skin of washed and unwashed hands and inoculating a plate of gelatin-like growth medium to characterize the growth of microorganisms that live on the skin during our daily lives. The fact that unwashed hands can transmit disease was discovered in the nineteenth century and is still one of the major ways that disease spreads.

In the mouth, salivary glands secrete mucus and proteins called immunoglobulins (*antibodies*) to trap and disable microorganisms that enter through the mouth or nose. Tears help wash away pathogens from the eyes. The acidity of the stomach is also able to kill many microorganisms before they can colonize the gut.

Immune function in the body has two "branches": the innate and adaptive immune systems. Often both work together to fight an infection. The innate immune system responds generally to invasion and to bacteria, viruses, and parasites and does not need to be pre-exposed to a disease. The adaptive immune system recognizes particular bacteria, viruses, and parasites and generates an active response to their presence.

The adaptive immune system is what is made use of by vaccination. This system recognizes infections that the body has already encountered and mounts a rapid defense against them, preventing illnesses from reestablishing infection once eliminated. The cell types of the adaptive immune system are subdivided into T and B cells.

B cells can be activated and have one of two fates. They can become plasma cells: factories that continuously produce antibodies, or they can become memory cells that "remember" a pathogen. When re-exposed to a pathogen, memory B cells can divide into plasma cells and more memory B cells.

Vaccines operate by placing in the body immune-generating structures that are not capable of causing disease on their own. These might be fragments of dead viruses or bacteria, a modified form of an organism that is less virulent, or a related organism that cannot infect humans. These create memory B cells, but do not create the disease. On first exposure to a pathogen, the immune system might take a week to ramp up production of antibodies. On a later exposure, its response will be more rapid and more specific, ramping up production of antibodies within hours. To someone who has been *immunized*, exposure to a disease such as smallpox has a lower chance of the disease progressing to symptoms because antibodies will be rapidly produced and the invader defeated.

In this way, vaccination is making use of the body's normal defenses by exposing them to nonpathogenic versions of normally disease-causing organisms. However, in the case of infectious diseases, vaccination is not just a process that happens to one person.

Imagine a hypothetical vaccine that reduces the likelihood of someone who has received it becoming sick when exposed to an infectious disease from 100 percent to 5 percent. The disease itself, once it has infected someone, will on average infect 10 more people. Imagine that the recipient of this vaccine lives in a village with 1,000 people; 10 of those 1,000 are immune compromised or too young to receive the vaccine. If only 1 vaccine were available, we might expect these people to become sick because they are unprotected. The disease would rapidly jump from 1 person to 10 people to 100 to 999. Soon the entire village would be sick.

If there were 800 vaccines available, you would expect about 240 people to become sick. These are those who were not vaccinated and those who were vaccinated but in whom the vaccine did not produce immunity. What happens if 950 vaccines are made available? If we extrapolate from the previous examples, we might expect that about 100 people would become sick, including those who are not vaccinated and those in whom the vaccine does not work. However, a phenomenon called *herd immunity* occurs when a large enough portion of a population is protected from a disease.

When enough of the population is protected from the disease, the incidence of the disease drops to the point where those who are vulnerable in the population are never exposed to it. Because infectious diseases survive by moving from one person to the next, if the disease cannot find a new host, it cannot continue. No one other than the initial patient (and perhaps one person with whom there is a chance encounter) becomes sick. Reaching this critical threshold in a population protects those who cannot receive a vaccine, which is why health officials often target vaccination rates to exceed herd-immunity thresholds. Once this threshold number exceeded, ongoing transmission of a disease can be ended. Efforts to eliminate diseases through vaccination rely on herd immunity to end transmission of infectious diseases.

The anti-vaccine movement is comprised of people who, for a variety of reasons, have chosen to oppose vaccination. Often the movement is attributed solely to developments as recent as the late 1990s, but its origins go back much further to the origins of vaccination itself. Understanding how early anti-vaccine movements arose, as well as the arguments they made, will help us understand the modern anti-vaccine movement because many of the arguments and motivations behind it have not changed.

3   The World before Vaccines

Upon a general calculation, threescore persons in every hundred have the small-pox. Of these threescore, twenty die of it in the most favourable season of life, and as many more wear the disagreeable remains of it in their faces so long as they live. Thus, a fifth part of mankind either die or are disfigured by this distemper.

—Voltaire[1]

To those of us raised in the latter half of the twentieth century or the early part of the twenty-first, it is astonishing that in the eighteenth century it was an inevitable fact of life that you were more likely to die from communicable diseases[2] than from today's leading causes of death, cardiovascular disease and cancer. In the world of the late eighteenth century, infectious disease was an inevitable feature of everyday life. The life expectancy at birth in England in 1750 was approximately thirty-five years.[3] This low life expectancy was exacerbated by what is today an unthinkable infant-mortality rate. So-called puerperal fever,[4] a postchildbirth infection often spread by physicians, took many lives, and preeclampsia, hemorrhage, and cephalopelvic disproportion were not understood, or well treated, making birth a significant risk for the mother, as well as the child. A life without major infectious illness was a luxurious rarity.

The bubonic plague periodically killed huge portions of the population of Europe, outbreaks of cholera and typhoid regularly occurred, and smallpox was ever present. Not only was disease rampant, but it wasn't understood. The discovery that diseases could be caused by microorganisms was a century in the future. Diseases were recognized and classified, but the medicine of the time at best was palliative and at worst did more harm than good. The first disease to be vaccinated against, and one of the first diseases to be investigated with an early version of the scientific method, was smallpox.

Smallpox was a disease with a 30 percent mortality rate, characterized by influenza-like symptoms followed by rashes and lesions on the skin and mucous membranes. Many survivors were left permanently scarred[5] or unable to see. Possibly at the time mortality rates were even higher because distinctions may not have been made between chickenpox and smallpox. It is believed that smallpox had blighted humanity since the earliest old world human agricultural civilizations, and characteristic lesions can be found even on preserved mummies from ancient Egypt.[6] Smallpox cared not for social class, intelligence, race, piety, or prayer. Smallpox was egalitarian in its reign of death and disfigurement, until it was made into a biological weapon in the genocide of Native Americans by Europeans. Unlike other diseases, such as malaria, smallpox was not limited by climate. When an immune population would grow old and die off, an epidemic would occur and once again kill and disfigure anew. Smallpox was nasty and miserable—not a fun time at all.

The disease gained its name, *variola*, from the same root as the English word "various," *varius* referring to the marks left upon the skin. Later the field of virology was developed, and it became possible to classify diseases based on characteristics of the agent that caused them, rather than the condition they produced. With smallpox, the condition was caused by a type of virus known as an orthopoxvirus.[7] Using modern methods, we now know that chickenpox, for example, belongs to a different family of viruses, despite carrying superficially similar symptoms, which is why the widespread vaccination for smallpox did not eliminate chickenpox.

There has not been a case of smallpox since the 1970s, and the only known samples exist in secure government research labs in the United States and Russia. The disease was declared eliminated on May 8, 1980. Diseases such as whooping cough and measles are now so rare as to be considered remarkable, and millions of dollars are spent every year researching ways to combat diseases such as malaria and HIV.

The idea that humans can, though focused effort, develop and arrive at *cures* for diseases is relatively modern. For most of our history the causes and mechanisms for disease were not understood. Medicine was prescientific and included such treatments as leeches and blood drawing for a variety of conditions.

One feature of smallpox that aided in attempts at its treatment is that once infected with smallpox, if a patient recovers, they are not later susceptible to the disease. Attempts were made to expose patients to smallpox as a way of preventing later infection in a process known as variolation. Variolation usually caused mild smallpox symptoms followed by a recovery. It is believed that the first variolation occurred in China or India, through a process of insufflation, whereby ground smallpox scabs or pustule fluid was inhaled through the nose,[8] and texts refer to a similar practice in India dating to the sixteenth century.[9] The practice did not make it into European medicine until 1714, although it was known by European physicians before that and commonly believed to be a folkloric treatment.[10]

Interestingly, the willingness of European physicians to ignore variolation mirrors later resistance to vaccination by some in the medical community. Regardless of when the practice entered the medical literature, there is evidence that it was widely known and practiced for a long time before its formalization in the early eighteenth century.[11] It is possible that the practice had multiple origins and is far older than recorded accounts; however, when it was practiced, it had a fairly low mortality rate and provided protection against smallpox. It did, however, carry risk. Those who were inoculated became carriers, who could then infect others with a full case of smallpox, and in a small number of cases, variolation led to a serious case of smallpox.

It may seem strange that a practice so widely employed wasn't accepted or known by the scientific and medical elite of the time. However, science at the time was in its infancy. Indeed the term *science* has had meanings that have shifted and changed through the centuries and probably still have not settled. In 1834 William Whewell was the first to use the term *scientist*,[12] by analogy to terms such as *artist*, to describe those who practice science. The Baconian method was first proposed in Francis Bacon's book *Novum Organum* in 1620. This was a landmark in the development of scientific reasoning for several reasons. It is one of the first times a systematic method for acquiring knowledge about the world based only on observed facts, rather than inference, was proposed. The structure of observation followed by hypothesis, followed by further observation is still important to the way that science is conducted today, although induction has been convincingly argued against as a sole means of acquiring scientific knowledge. In the seventeenth century, Newton, Leibniz, and Galileo were revolutionizing science. Descartes suggested a mechanical universe, and John Locke's writings influenced many to see knowledge as produced by human experience, rather than metaphysical inference. Antonie van Leeuwenhoek had used optics to discover that coexisting with the world we see and interact with there is another microscopic world full of what he called animalcules (tiny animals), which we now know were single-celled organisms. Yet the germ theory of disease would not gain acceptance for hundreds more years. Voltaire wrote about how those who practiced inoculation were viewed.

> It is inadvertently affirmed in the Christian countries of Europe that the English are fools and madmen. Fools, because they give their children the small-pox to prevent their catching it; and madmen, because they wantonly communicate a certain and dreadful distemper to their children, merely to prevent an uncertain evil.[13]

Science was gaining in influence, but the scientific methods that we now employ were not yet available. Statistical analysis was yet to emerge as a means of testing hypotheses, and the scientific norms such as journal publications and peer review did not yet exist. Often science proceeded in fits and starts by individual efforts, but science as a collective enterprise was not recognizable. Moreover, the concept of science as a career in which one might devote one's time to earning money was seen as unseemly. Those who studied science saw themselves as liberally educated and holding broad interests, including in the philosophy of the natural world.

This world of rampant disease, high infant mortality, and rising influence of scientific ideas is the background in which the first vaccine was discovered.

4 The First Vaccine

In science credit goes to the man who convinces the world, not the
man to whom the idea first occurs.

—Francis Galton

For most of the modern era of medicine, we have considered
viruses to be nonliving. A virus is a fragment of genetic material
called RNA, or DNA encapsulated by a coat of protein, which
may sometimes be modified by fats or sugars. Of the things that
most scientists agree are characteristic of living things, viruses
only exhibit a few. They do not metabolize, grow, or generally
respond to stimulus. They do reproduce, but only by infecting
cells and hijacking their machinery, which normally replicates
RNA and DNA and produces proteins. Viruses evolve, like living
things, but because they are obligate parasites with no independent lifecycle, they are viewed as living.

DNA and RNA are molecules whose main function is to carry
information in a stable and copyable manner. A sugar backbone
holds interchangeable molecules, the sequence of which can be
interpreted by the machinery of the cell to produce specific proteins. Proteins are also long chains built Lego-like from a limited

number of molecules. The genetic material of a virus tells the cell which proteins to make to produce more viruses and is duplicated into every individual viral particle produced by an infected cell. These duplications are often imperfect and introduce errors into the viruses produced by that cell; these errors are known as mutations.

The two most common fates for mutated viruses are either that the mutant has no change in its ability to infect cells and reproduce or that it becomes less efficient or unable to reproduce. These mutations are less "fit" to reproduce and do not survive. Rarely, but occasionally, a mutation increases the ability of a virus to infect some cell types and reproduce more. Because these viruses are a better fit to their environment, they enjoy easier reproduction and therefore will often outcompete their less well-adapted counterparts. Viruses will often evolve along divergent paths and with different strains to become better fits to different environments, such as different host species or cell types.

Smallpox shares an evolutionary ancestor with another virus known as cowpox. Cowpox infects the udders of cows and produces lesions similar to those of smallpox. It is also *zoonotic*, meaning it can be transmitted between humans and nonhuman animals. Because humans are not its primary host, cowpox presents much milder symptoms to infected humans than does smallpox and is generally not lethal to humans. Another important feature of cowpox is that it shares molecular similarities with smallpox and looks very similar to smallpox to the human immune system.

This information about viruses was unknown in the late eighteenth century, but in 1768 the surgeon John Fewster started a practice with a local inoculator and made an observation:

some people, although repeatedly exposed to smallpox, did not develop any symptoms, despite never having had the disease. As an explanation, a farmer suggested to him, "I have had the Cowpox lately to a violent degree, if that's any odds." Investigating, Fewster discovered that all those whom he could not inoculate with smallpox had at some point had cowpox. He did not, however, see the point of using cowpox as a substitute in variolation, as he believed smallpox inoculation to be well understood.[1]

> Remember kids, the only difference between screwing around and science is writing it down.
> —Alex Jason, often attributed to Adam Savage

Another reason that Fewster is not credited with the discovery of vaccination is that although he made the initial observation and reported it, he did not undertake in a systematic way to test it. In fact, several people recorded attempts to use cowpox as a means to inoculate against smallpox. Peter Plett, a German teacher, was probably the first to recognize the importance of the discovery and reported his findings to the medical faculty at the University of Kiel. Those faculty favored variolation, so the report was never forwarded.[2] Plett is rarely credited.

Indeed, as many as six people before Jenner, who is most often credited with the discovery of vaccination, made this observation. Although we think of scientific discoveries as belonging to individuals, it is often the case that attributing appropriate credit is messy and difficult. Jenner was the first to popularize the discovery and is therefore given credit for it. For many discoveries, credit is hotly debated, as in the cases of Rosalind Franklin, whose contributions to the discovery of the structure of DNA were not recognized until after her death, and Jocelyn

Bell Burnell, who as a postgraduate student made observations
that led to the discovery of pulsars but was not included in the
Nobel prize awarded for it to her thesis supervisor and other
authors of the paper.

The stage was set for Jenner's work on vaccines by a number
of figures and discoveries that occurred in the seventeenth century. Lady Mary Wortley Montagu is credited with introducing
the practice of variolation to England. Although she cannot be
said to have discovered variolation, she traveled to what is now
Turkey and wrote to a friend about variolation being used in
the Ottoman court. Upon returning to England, Lady Montagu
introduced variolation to the royal physician, who then experimented on six prisoners in 1721, on the promise of a full pardon. This experiment was observed by members of the Royal
Society. Later he experimented on six orphans in London, and
finally on the children of the princess of Wales.

Human experimentation (as was also performed by Jenner)
was not at the time governed by the same ethical rules that it is
now. Today, offering pardon in exchange for being a subject to a
potentially deadly experimental treatment or experimenting on
children would be seen as hideously unethical and would never
pass review.

The first recorded intentional vaccination with cowpox
occurred two decades before Jenner's work. Benjamin Jesty, a
farmer, used cowpox to vaccinate his family. In 1774 smallpox
was noted near his farm. He used a darning needle, exposed to
pus from an infected cow, to scratch his wife and children. Their
wounds became inflamed, but all survived. Later, in 1789, his
children were inoculated with smallpox but did not display a
reaction.[3] According to a physician who wrote of the attempt
in 1803, "The boldness and novelty of the attempt produced no

small alarm in the family, and no small sensation in the neighbourhood."[4] The inflammation of his wife's arm produced such upset that a neighboring surgeon almost lost his practice when proposing a follow-up experiment to Jesty's. There was objection to "introducing the bestial disorder to the human frame." Jesty was credited with resisting the "clamorous reproaches of his neighbors."

Remarkably, this first recorded instance of vaccination also marked the first recorded instance of opposition to vaccination, although in this case the reasoning behind the opposition was likely sound. With no medical training or equipment, Jesty had used a darning needle to infect his family with pus from a cow's diseased udder, an experiment resulting in an alarming infection. This was also the first instance of what would become a running theme in history: revulsion and visceral horror at the mere notion polluting one's body with alien materials. Concerns about safety and fear of taking foreign material into the body often still characterize anti-vaccination rhetoric two hundred and fifty years after Jesty's "bold" experiment.

Ultimately, Edward Jenner was credited with the discovery of vaccination because he was the first to systematically test the idea that exposure to cowpox would prevent later smallpox infection. During his childhood, Jenner was inoculated against smallpox. He became a physician, and before his work on vaccines, he was elected to the Royal Society, the most important scientific body of the time in England, for a study of cuckoos, showing that when cuckoos laid eggs in the nests of other birds, it was not the parent cuckoo who ejected the eggs of the parasitized birds from their nests but the newly hatched cuckoo. Fellowship in the Royal Society was among the era's greatest scientific honors.

Jenner began with an understanding that domestication of animals had exposed humans to animal diseases and that certain infections could be transmitted from animals to humans.[5] He then made essentially the same observation that others before him had: that milkmaids who had contracted cowpox did not react to inoculation with a reduced course of smallpox infection. This observation led to the formation of a hypothesis: that inoculation with cowpox acted similarly to inoculation with smallpox, to provide protection against later smallpox infection. Jenner meticulously collected case reports that seemed to support the idea. He asked his inoculation patients if they had ever had cowpox, and he recorded the results of inoculation with smallpox, observing that consistently those patients who were exposed to smallpox were unaffected by cowpox, and vice versa.

The distinguishing feature that Jenner brought to vaccination was a systematic attempt to collect individual anecdotes. This is more scientific than a single, unreported experiment, as Benjamin Jesty tried on his family. Happening at the dawn of the scientific era, vaccination grew up at the same time that science did. Jenner also relied on human experimentation in a way that would not be permitted today. He learned the scientific method as "Why think—why not try the experiment?"[6] After assuring himself that the folk wisdom of cowpox preventing later infection by smallpox was true, he did the experiment. In May 1796, Sarah Nelmes, a dairymaid, was infected with cowpox in a scratch on her hand. Jenner then found a healthy boy of about eight years old to experiment on.

> The matter was taken from a sore on the hand of a dairymaid, who was infected by her master's cows and it was inserted, on the 14th of May, 1796 into the arm of the boy by means of two superficial incisions, barely penetrating the cutis,[7] each about half an inch long.[8]

After the infection with cowpox ran its course, Jenner inoculated the boy with smallpox from a fresh pustule on July 1, 1796. The weak case of smallpox normally observed after inoculation did not occur. Several months later Jenner tried again to infect the boy and found similar results. If it seems unethical to experimentally infect healthy children with deadly diseases to satisfy one's personal curiosity, it is. The best that can be said, without excusing the behavior, is that Jenner would likely have inoculated the boy with smallpox regardless of his experiment. Inoculation was a practice Jenner was very familiar with and believed he could do safely, despite the procedure's (low) mortality rate. He knew cowpox to be nonfatal, so the minor suffering of cowpox seemed to him worth the possibility of avoiding the roughly 3 percent risk of death from variolation.

At this point, Jenner was delayed for two years as he was unable to refrigerate or store viruses until cowpox infections were once again available. In March 1798 he inoculated two five-year-old children. One became sick with a fever that Jenner attributed to the child's being in a workhouse. The other provided material to inoculate another boy, who displayed a fever consistent with smallpox but not the pustules. Emboldened, in April, Jenner inoculated several more children with cowpox. Most of these cowpox inoculations were followed with attempts to inoculate these patients with smallpox. The name Jenner gave to this process was "vaccination," from the Latin word *vacca*, meaning cow.

Opposition to the idea of vaccination was swift. Jenner's original paper was rejected by the Royal Society as being too fantastical and in opposition to what was previously known,[9] but he published his results in a booklet.[10] Jenner's work was seen not only as blurring the line between human and beast but between social classes. It was shocking that information gleaned from pastoral farmers and milkmaids might advance medical science, which was considered to be the domain of the educated elite.[11] Those with economic interests in variolation were especially doubtful of the new technology.

> Can any person say what may be the consequences of introducing a bestial humour into the human frame, after a long lapse of years? Who knows besides, what ideas may rise, in the course of time, from a brutal fever having excited its incongruous impression on the brain. Who knows, also, that the human character may undergo strange mutations from quadruped sympathy; and that some modern Pasiphae[12] may rival the fables of old?
>
> —Benjamin Moseley[13]

As vaccination gained traction, so did opposition to it. Pamphlets were distributed opposing vaccination and comparing it to opposing Napoleon's army. Vaccination was framed as a foreign assault on traditional order. However, this early opposition was recognized as hyperbolic and rejected by the medical community. Jenner shrewdly began an influence campaign. He met with the king, the prince, and finally the queen of the United Kingdom, using their approval to speed adoption among the aristocracy, from whom it spread to their tenants. Jenner made a political decision to ally himself with establishment forces in order to speed the adoption of vaccination.

Adoption of vaccination was not immediate in the medical community, but by 1840 it had supplanted variolation, which was outlawed in England with the British Vaccination Act of 1840. In part this was triggered by the news of an 1837 outbreak of smallpox carried by fur traders into the American West. More than 17,000 people died (possibly double this number), many of them Native Americans. A full accounting was never made because at some point the bodies could no longer be counted. Over the following century, the act of 1840 and a series of laws passed in 1853, 1867, 1871, 1873, 1889, 1898, and 1907 laid out UK policy regarding vaccines. The act of 1840 provided optional free vaccination in addition to outlawing variolation.[14] Importantly, this created a public vaccination service, which survived for decades. The act of 1853 triggered the first formal, organized opposition to vaccination.

5   The First Anti-vaccine Movements

Early opposition to vaccination was intimately tied to issues of social class, individual liberties, individual and collective rights, and changing ideas about health and medicine. While many disliked the idea of vaccination in its first decades, organized opposition to the practice of vaccination was not common until the British government began mandating it.

Because the Vaccination Act of 1853 required mandatory vaccination for all infants over four months old, it raised issues of civil liberties and numerous civic and religious concerns—about bearing the costs of vaccination for the poor,[1] about placing material from cows into humans, about preserving the integrity of the body, and about disrupting the "natural order." Those who believed in the power of vaccination to improve human health and well-being and in the right of the state to impose vaccination found themselves in a war of both information and culture.

The philosophy of health for many simply did not include scientific experimentation or analysis. The emerging field of science-based medicine was in competition with "alternative" approaches, such as homeopathy, heroic medicine,[2] and "folk medicine." Absent the rigor of experimental and scientific approaches to understanding disease, such alternative approaches were appealing. Indeed, even those administering vaccines in that era did so in a way that we would now consider to be unsanitary, painful, and sometimes disfiguring. Pus would be taken with a tool called a lancet from a pustule of one vaccinated individual and used to vaccinate the next. Colonial powers would impose vaccination on unwilling populations. Vaccine material would be collected from sores on infants who had recently been vaccinated. These practices possibly transmitted other communicable diseases.

At the time poorer economic classes often did not have access to clean water or wound care, and secondary infections could develop from vaccination. Those who believed that health was maintained through integrity of the body saw compulsory vaccination as an outrageous overreach of the state into personal affairs. Those living in colonies of the era often saw vaccination as just another means for controlling and dominating the population. A person's body was the last battleground, where individual liberties would face off against the growing authority of the state.

During the same century, a series of acts seemed to assert the rights of the state over the bodies of especially the poor and women. The Anatomy Act of 1832—which was intended to prevent the shortage of available bodies for dissection and the study of anatomy—expanded the range of usable corpses from only those of executed murderers to those whose remains were never claimed; and, in the view of many, the act allowed the wealthy to dissect the poor. The Contagious Disease Acts required medical inspection of those suspected of prostitution, in order to look for venereal disease, regardless of their consent.

Much of the prevalent anti-vaccine sentiment of the era was laid out in 1854, when John Gibbs, esquire, published the booklet *Our medical liberties, or The personal rights of the subject, as infringed by recent and proposed legislation: compromising observations on the compulsory vaccination act, the medical registration and reform bills, and the Maine laws.* He was in favor of neither compulsory vaccination nor short titles.

Gibbs attacked the Vaccination Act of 1853 on several fronts, complaining that it was an intrusion on personal rights, that it was written to benefit the medical trade, that it treated the populous as too stupid to make their own health decisions, that it mandated a practice that was not universally accepted among physicians, and that it had failed in some individual cases.[3] The similarity of his pamphlet's arguments to those made by modern vaccine opponents is striking. Gibbs went on to make a much weaker argument in the light of modern scientific knowledge. He argued that the fundamental nature of human biology (and therefore of disease) changed intermittently and that scientific studies of disease were therefore useless. He argued that vaccination, regardless of its protective effects against smallpox might have "influence generally upon the constitution. … Does it lower the vital resistance and predispose the system to receive or does it introduce it to other forms of disease?" His complaint that vaccination benefited the medical trade may have been related to his own occupation as in hydropathy,[4] a kind of quack medicine that involved treatment by bathing in, drinking, or injecting water and applying it to various parts of the body. Given the hygiene practices of the era, promoting bathing was, perhaps, not the worst idea that he had, but it was not an effective means of preventing smallpox infection. A similar tension exists today. Science-based medicine exerts a monopoly on the treatment of disease, and at its periphery "alternative" practitioners market non-evidence-based approaches to health care.

At the same time as vaccination was developing, so was the new science of statistics.[5] In the modern era, statistics is its own mathematical science with a number of well-understood methods and ways of formalizing results. Statistics started as a way for states to collect information about the populations living in them for analysis. The fundamental problem statistics solves is that it is difficult or impossible to survey every member of a population for every parameter you might want to test. For example, if you want to know how many men wear hats in the United States, you could survey every man in the United States, or you could attempt to get an estimate by surveying a subset of men. Statistics allows us to decide how many men to survey, how likely our results are to represent the entire US population, and how much we should trust our results based on that data.

The development of probability theory allowed for the use of testing hypotheses by statistical means. There is a possibility, for example, that if you pick ten American men at random to survey, you have had the bad luck of picking ten hat wearers, or ten non–hat wearers, by random chance. Statistics allows us to estimate the probability of having a representative sample. It also allows us to estimate the likelihood that two measured groups are different because of random chance, rather than an actual difference. If we sample ten people from New York and ten from San Antonio and find ten hat wearers in New York and only five in San Antonio, statistics will allow us to know if we have sampled enough people from each city to draw a reasonable conclusion.

However, statistics can be deployed badly, or in bad faith. The often complex-looking equations and symbols of statistics can be used to communicate quickly and succinctly between those with statistical training, and they can be used to confuse, befuddle, and bully into belief those without. Gibbs's booklet provides examples of the latter approach. By selecting only data that seemed to support his views, a kind of bias that scientists often call cherry picking, he could imply alarming trends. A rise in death rates due to measles in specific cities can be attributed to vaccination by means of a confusion between correlation and causation. These same means of misrepresenting statistical information are still used today by modern anti-vaccine activists.

To understand the reaction to the Vaccination Act of 1853, we need to consider it in its political context. John Locke's writings on natural rights were still influential at the time. Locke proposed that what he called "natural rights," as distinct from legal rights, were rights belonging to every human that could not be altered by human laws. Locke identified these as life, liberty, and property.

An alternative view, also circulating at the time, was proposed by Jean-Jacques Rousseau in *The Social Contract*. Rousseau proposed that the right of people to be governed should come from agreement between the government and the governed, rather than from divine mandate. Everyone ought to give up the same rights to government and assume the same duties. Thomas Hobbes supported this line of thought, arguing that if humans are born with the natural rights to take any actions, those rights lead to a "war against all" to compete for resources and safety. Therefore, humans must give up most rights in order to live among other humans.

It was in this background of competing ideas about the rights of individuals and the rights of collectives in the form of government that these early vaccine objections occurred. We still debate the boundaries between individual and collective rights today, and these debates inform our modern political philosophies and motivations.

Setting aside the question of whether the government had a right to impose vaccination, Gibbs brought forth the question of whether vaccination worked, which was easier to answer with the emerging fields of science and mathematics. Success had recently been had in using science to prevent cholera. The Public Health Act of 1848 was created to combat cholera epidemics, by improving sanitation and the supply of water, and establish a General Board of Health to oversee local boards of health. These boards would take over public sewers, purchase private sewers, institute street cleaning, provide public lavatories, and supply water. This process was pioneered by John Simon, a surgeon who was appointed as the medical officer of health for London, chief medical officer of the General Board of Health, and later chief medical officer to the Privy Council. Simon was a strong advocate for vaccination and presented a strong rebuttal to claims by anti-vaccine activists that vaccination did not work. Simon wrote:

> Hence, in the middle of the 19th century, the very success of vaccination may have blinded people it its importance. It is so easy to be bold against an absent danger—to despise the antidote while one has no painful experience of the bane.[6]

Simon presented to parliament and the queen papers making an extended argument in favor of vaccination. He detailed the history of its opposition, commenting, "It is wearisome work to read stuff so stupid or so dishonest," in response to claims that vaccines were causing people to become cow-like, burst forth with horns, or behave in a beastly manner. He also pointed out that disagreements in the medical profession tended to amplify dissenting voices, but, by and large, the opinions of the medical profession had been fixed since the earliest part of the nineteenth century. Remarkably, he made a statistical argument, not only that vaccination had reduced deaths by smallpox tenfold to twentyfold (figure 5.1) but that in the exceptional cases where vaccination did not prevent later disease, the severity of the disease was likely to be mitigated. He cited work by a surgeon from a London smallpox hospital showing a fatality rate of 35 percent in the unvaccinated, and 0.5 percent in the vaccinated. Furthermore, he showed that revaccination worked to protect

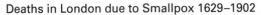

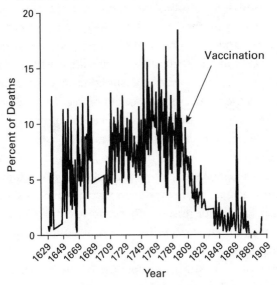

Figure 5.1

Deaths in London due to smallpox, 1629–1902: The discovery and popularization of vaccination preceded a sharp decline in the number of deaths in London. Historical records in other nations don't all go as far back, but all show a similar decline coinciding with the introduction of vaccination. Countries with mandatory vaccination programs showed sharper declines than those without. (Adapted from W. A. Guy, "Two Hundred and Fifty Years of Small Pox in London," *Journal of the Statistical Society of London* 45 [1882]: 399.)

the majority of those who had once again become susceptible. Debunking the idea that vaccination itself was causing harm, Simon showed that the overall death rate had declined in the years since the discovery of vaccination.

However, Simon made a mistake that has become frequent among vaccine advocates. He focused only on the scientific challenges that denialists offered and did not make an effort to address the true underlying reasons for their concerns.

Gibbs and other anti-vaccine activists did not make scientific objections because they had approached the question with an open mind, and through scientific inquiry, they had decided that vaccination was ineffective. They started with a complex network of personal reasons for objecting to vaccination and approached the science as a source of prestige that could be borrowed for their arguments. From this viewpoint no experiment can be well enough designed, no controls adequate, and no evidence convincing. The effectiveness of vaccination was beside the point—a mere rhetorical tool to be wielded by whomever was most convincing. The theme of anti-vaccine advocates reaching their conclusions for reasons other than scientific analysis and not changing their views in the face of scientific evidence is a recurring one.

Simon was a member and founder of the Epidemiological Society of London, founded to *"venienti occurrite morbo,"* or confront disease at its onset.[7] The society had a bold mandate: to use the developing tools of science to study epidemics and come to a better understanding of their origins and causes. This society signaled a shift in belief about disease, from seeing it a mysterious force that was largely outside of human control to seeing it as a natural and mechanical phenomenon that could be analyzed and understood. One of the society's founders, John

Snow, famously used statistics in 1854 to study the Broad Street cholera outbreak, which killed thirty-one thousand Londoners. By treating the water with chlorine and removing the handle of the water pump that was the source of the infection, he ended the epidemic. This work convincingly showed that cholera is waterborne and not caused by miasma,[8] and was chronicled in the 2006 book *The Ghost Map* by Steven Johnson. In the same year, an Italian physician observed small organisms living in cholera-causing water, which he believed to transmit the disease by acting on the intestine. His theory was later proved correct, as was his proposed treatment of injection with electrolytes and water to supplement losses due to diarrhea.

The Epidemiological Society of London was symbolic of two trends, one toward the professionalization of medicine and another toward the development of medicine as an applied science. The distinctions among natural scientists, formal scientists, social scientists, and applied scientists had not yet been made in the minds of most who did scientific work or in the mind of the public. Broadly speaking, a natural science is a science that studies the natural world and seeks to understand its underlying rules and mechanisms, while an applied science applies knowledge gained through scientific methods to solving problems in the world. However, the idea that medicine should be based on only that which can be experimentally verified was novel. Those who claimed to cure and treat diseases practiced without licensure and might use any number of methods and modalities.

The idea of a physician as a member of a professional class was unusual. It seemed to be a way for those with the means to take even more away from common people. In many ways these objections were well founded. In the early nineteenth century, the physicians who would evolve into being members of the medical profession we now recognize were little better than quacks and offered a variety of services and cures that we now recognize as being abject nonsense.

Professionalization provided a means to control not only who could call themselves physicians and administer treatments but also the quality of those treatments and the means of deciding how to use them. When the Vaccination Act of 1853 was being considered, the Epidemiological Society of London had a great deal of influence on its creation. Rather than known community members administering variolation, in an often ritualistic and comforting setting, strangers, asserting the authority of the state, were performing a *procedure*. Given the condition of the medical profession in the early nineteenth century— riddled with pseudoscience and quack practitioners—a primary motivator of this professionalization was the desire for return on investment.[9] Why pay for medical school if someone with no education could practice just as easily? The Medical Act of 1858 established a council for the education and registration of medical practitioners. This granted medicine one of the central features of a profession: self-regulation.[10] To this day, some see the requirement that healers be educated as an unfair imposition that creates a monopoly. The alternative are treatments that have not met the standards of scientific rigor and reproducibility necessary to being considered medicine.

A side effect of professionalization was the development of professional ethics. Professional ethics is a means by which medical practitioners can exert influence and control over the behaviors of their peers in line with an agreed-upon code of ethics. To this day, medical ethics are influenced by the work of Thomas Percival, who first published *Medical Ethics* in 1803, where he wrote:

The *feelings* and *emotions* of the patients, under critical circumstances, require to be known and attended to, no less than the symptoms of their diseases.[11]

Social and political class divides in the era of Victorian England were stark. Thomas Malthus had published in 1798 *An Essay on the Principle of Population*, which proposed a troubling idea. In essence he argued that populations tended to grow in size over time. Because populations grow they must consume more resources over time. But given that certain resources are limited, Malthus proposed that so long as population growth continues, the scarcity of resources would cause ever greater poverty, until the incentives to have more children were reduced and the population once again stabilized. In his view populations would oscillate between growth, when new resources became available, and a stable equilibrium, when not.[12] Among Malthus's suggested solutions was the proposal of the elimination of social programs aiding the poor. If the poverty were so miserable that it was not possible to reproduce, he reasoned, fewer poor people would have children.

Malthus's idea was deeply influential, as were those of David Ricardo, published in *On the Principles of Political Economy and Taxation* (1817), which argued that taxes raised for the relief of poverty reduced funds available to pay wages and encouraged laziness. Another influential thinker was Jeremy Bentham. Bentham was an early advocate for women's rights, abolition of slavery, abolition of the death penalty, animal rights, and gay rights. He was also an atheist, who opposed the idea of natural rights as granted by a divine power and therefore disliked the American Declaration of Independence, which borrowed heavily from Locke's ideas. Bentham's major philosophical stance is known as utilitarianism, which is the view that the moral rightness of an act depends on its doing the most good for the most people. Bentham also believed that free markets should set wages and that collecting taxes to relieve the poor interfered with the free market.[13]

With these new ideas influencing the thinking of legislators, plans were made to alter the way the government dealt with poverty and disease. The Poor Law Amendment Act of 1834 changed how the poor were provided relief. Rather than being given money and allowed to choose how to spend it themselves, those unable to find work would need to go to a workhouse, where manual labor could be traded for food and clothing under what we would now consider to be cruel, prison-like conditions,[14] with harsh discipline that separated families and encouraged child labor. The Poor Law Amendment Act also consolidated local control of poverty relief at that parish level to larger unions overseen by Boards of Guardians.[15] Within a year several of the unions had to deal with riots and significant unrest. Laborers began to organize marches, and officials representing workhouses were assaulted, but the opposition was disorganized and fell apart within a few months. Some, seeing an opportunity, began campaigns to organize opposition. The Reverend F. H. Maberly distributed leaflets and organized meetings with as many as two thousand attendees in an attempt to raise opposition to the new system but ultimately failed to start a sustained movement. However, later in the 1830s, when unions began implementing the new Poor Law in the north, organizers experienced with opposition to factory conditions, who emerged from trade unionism and factory-reform movements, would later become leaders in opposition to vaccination. The leaders who emerged from trade unionism and factory-reform movements would later become leaders in opposition to vaccination.

Given the unrest that followed the Poor Laws, as well as the generally poor understanding of the nature of smallpox vaccination, it should be unsurprising that many who opposed the Poor Laws also opposed mandatory vaccination. Not only did the methods developed in opposing the Poor Laws adapt to opposition to the vaccination act, the act itself was seen by many as another salvo in a war against the poor, taking away from them the last dignity they were afforded: control of their own bodies.

"Alternative" medical practitioners attacked the professionalizing system of medicine, both out of fear of losing market share and because medicine at the time was hardly effective[16] and benefited those elites who could afford advanced education. These practitioners led the early opposition of vaccination—as was the case with Gibbs's pamphlet. The circulation of the pamphlet led to a letter sent to the board of health in 1855, "Compulsory Vaccination Briefly Considered in Its Scientific, Religious and Political Aspects." This pamphlet repeated many of Gibbs's arguments and was widely distributed.

In 1866 the first organized opposition to vaccination formed, the Anti-Compulsory Vaccination League (ACVL), organized by John Gibbs's cousin Richard Butler Gibbs, modeled on previous reform movements. Within a few years, it had over one hundred chapters. The ACVL published journals, issued memberships, and of course accepted donations. Although these organizations claimed to act against vaccination on behalf of the working class, the membership was often decidedly middle-class. A number of similar groups arose and began the work of distributing handbills, pamphlets, photographs, and magic-lantern slides of vaccine wound sites. In 1867 and the early 1870s, a series of additional vaccination acts were passed, in response to the growing anti-vaccination movement. These acts updated the process by which vaccination was to be carried out and reaffirmed that vaccination was to be compulsory.

According to one history of the era, *Bodily Matters: The Anti-Vaccination Movement in England, 1853–1907*,[17] many Victorians looked on anti-vaccine activists as fringe cranks, lumping it with other contemporary movements. Indeed, anti-vaccine activists found support in trade unions, among religious nonconformists, and among alternative medical practitioners. Vaccination took on a decidedly anti-establishment character.

By the 1880s it became common among anti-vaccine activists to attack and harass public health officials. In 1885 the most massive march of the anti-vaccine movement occurred in Leicester. A particular point of contention was the punishments being enforced against five thousand people who had refused vaccination.[18] Demonstrators came from many towns and cities[19] and may have had up to one hundred thousand attendees.

As in many towns, in Leicester, the growth of the population exceeded the capacity of sanitary arrangements and drainage. After the 1872–1873 smallpox epidemic left over three hundred people dead and the Vaccination Act of 1871 made vaccination compulsory, many saw the practice of vaccination as unnecessary, as it had in their view failed to protect those killed in the epidemic.[20] In the period leading up to the 1885 riots, over sixty Leicester residents were jailed for noncompliance with vaccination. Leicester developed its own methods of dealing with smallpox by isolating the infected; cleaning, disinfecting, or burning clothes and bedding; and similarly isolating those who had been in contact with the sick. Vaccination became an issue in municipal elections, and by 1884 the vaccination rate had dropped to 36 percent from 86 percent in 1873, largely due to the efforts of anti-vaccine activists. In late March delegates from the anti-vaccination leagues of over fifty towns arrived in Leicester. On the March 23 a crowd gathered at the Temperance Hall and marched with flags and banners to the marketplace, where they heard speeches.

In 1879 William Tebb, a prominent British anti-vaccine activist, visited New York City. Soon after, the Anti-Vaccination Society of America was founded, quickly followed by the New England Anti–Compulsory Vaccination League and the Anti-Vaccination League of New York City.[21] These groups were successful in repealing compulsory vaccination laws in a number of states. In 1905 the US Supreme Court ruled on *Jacobson v. Massachusetts* over a five-dollar fine imposed on a pastor who refused to vaccinate. The court ruled that states may restrict individual liberties if great dangers to the safety of the general public are present.[22] A concession was made, however: although states could punish those who refuse to vaccinate with fines or imprisonment, they could not forcibly vaccinate. The ruling also required that a medical exemption be made available for those who for whatever reason were medically unfit to be vaccinated. An analogy was made to periods of wartime, when individual liberties may be reduced in order to protect the larger community. This case marked an establishment of a legal balance between the rights of an individual and those of the collective.

By 1898 in the United Kingdom, a new vaccination act gave victory to anti-vaccine activists in the form of an option for conscientious objectors to avoid vaccination, essentially both handing a victory to the anti-vaccination movement and causing a loss of interest in it.

Other countries handled smallpox differently. The publication of Jenner's research coincided with a time when England was preparing to be invaded. France initially treated vaccination as a military technology, which would allow soldiers to avoid sickness, but did not require compulsory vaccination of the citizenry Vaccinators did begin the work of vaccination, however, and the fifty thousand to eighty thousand annual deaths due to smallpox in France were reduced to one-tenth of their previous level by 1850.[23]

Anti-vaccine activism was by no means limited to England and the United States. In 1904 Dr. Oswaldo Cruz convinced the Congress in Brazil to make vaccination mandatory. The use of force to enforce the law was not well received. An anti-vaccination league was formed and within five days began recruiting. After ten days violence broke out and riots ensued. Thirty people died, and over one hundred were injured. A general attempted to march on the presidential palace. The government relented, at least temporarily. Nevertheless, in 1908 a smallpox epidemic killed nine thousand people living in Rio de Janeiro.

Contemporaneous with the first anti-vaccine movements, the first steps toward the fields of microbiology and bacteriology were taken. Louis Pasteur developed the first theory of microorganisms as playing a role in metabolic processes and in 1858 published these results. He discovered that microorganisms were the cause of spoilage in food and drink and that heating (pasteurization) could be used to prevent the transmission of disease by infected milk. Joseph Lister became aware of this work and began experimenting with the use of solutions of phenol to prevent the spread of gangrene in wounds and developed methods of chemically sterilizing surgical instruments that greatly reduced the rate of infection. These discoveries helped the germ theory of disease displace other ideas about the causes of disease, such as the miasma theory. Under the germ theory of disease, many diseases are caused by microorganisms.[1]

The development of sterilization and the realization that microorganisms were responsible for causing many diseases also led to improvements in the ways that vaccines were transmitted, stored, and administered. In 1850 glycerol had been used as a means of storing vaccine matter, called lymph, for longer periods of time while still remaining effective, but the discovery was not widely disseminated or used until later in the nineteenth century.[2] In the early twentieth century, it was discovered that this effect also reduced the bacterial count within the lymph,[3] thus making it safer and less likely to produce unintended infections in patients. Another innovation was the inoculation of cow flanks to produce vaccine lymph because this method was less likely to transmit infections from human host to human host than was collecting lymph from humans.[4] Refrigeration allowed for longer-term storage of the lymph. In the 1950s means of freeze drying virus mixed with a protein called peptone were developed.[5] This allowed much longer-term storage at ambient temperatures without degradation. Over time several alternative methods of producing vaccine material were discovered, other than incubation on cow skin, such as incubation in eggs and in cells grown in dishes. Interestingly, the virus we now have that is used to produce smallpox vaccine, vaccinia, is of unknown origin. Vaccinia is related to, but not identical with, the cowpox virus; has been transmitted through replication in laboratories over many generations; and may be more closely related to horsepox, which was also used in the nineteenth century for vaccination.[6]

During the late nineteenth century Pasteur was also very active in investigating the nature of microbial life. At the time, the prevailing theory of the origins of life was spontaneous generation. Under this view, certain conditions were naturally appropriate for life to arise, and it would appear when those appropriate conditions arose. For example, spoiled meat was thought to naturally generate flies, and broth was thought to naturally generate bacteria when left unattended. In 1862 Pasteur showed that by preventing microorganisms from gaining entry to boiled broth it would not become cloudy with growth. Later Pasteur developed the second effective vaccine in history, which protected against anthrax. He had earlier shown that anthrax is caused by a bacterium.[7] By isolating and then using chemicals to attenuate, or reduce the infectivity of, the anthrax bacterium, he was able to develop a vaccine that provides immunity to anthrax with a significantly reduced chance of infection.[8] In 1885 he had the first successful human test of a vaccine he had developed against rabies, again using a method of attenuation. Attenuation of vaccines by various means continues to be used in various forms to this day.

At the end of the Victorian era, sporadic outbreaks of smallpox still occurred. In 1885 Montreal became subject to one such outbreak. A much smaller epidemic had been occurring between 1876 and 1880, but civil authorities did little.[9] The virus was brought to Montreal by an infected person on a railcar, and Boston had a minor outbreak from the same railcar but acted swiftly to vaccinate, so only six people in the city were infected. The civil authorities in Montreal were unprepared and slow at obtaining the vaccine. When news came out that vaccination was to be made mandatory, anti-vaccination rhetoric had been so effective that a "mob" of several thousand people congregated and took possession of the streets. The group wrecked the Health Office, and threw stones through the windows of physicians and the city health officer. Order was eventually restored, but a skirmish erupted with Canadian cavalry which only ended when they were ordered to load their rifles. Although this was the last major outbreak of smallpox in a city in the developed world, it would be nearly another century before smallpox was wiped out completely. The citizens of Montreal bought into anti-vaccine rhetoric and in doing so left themselves open to infection. While other cities had occasional occurrences of smallpox, the vaccination rate was high enough to prevent an epidemic.

The very fact that smallpox outbreaks became remarkable is itself remarkable. Figure 5.1 shows the incidence of smallpox in London between 1629 and 1902 as a percentage of deaths. Before the discovery of vaccination, smallpox was responsible for a little under 10 percent of deaths in London, dropping to less than 5 percent by the 1850s, with the exception of a pandemic in 1870. It is difficult to estimate the number of lives saved by a technology such as smallpox vaccination. Even a few decades before its eradication, 10 to 15 million people were newly infected, and 1.5 to 2 million human beings died annually,[10] especially in the developing world. An estimated 300 million people died of smallpox in the twentieth century alone, as if the entire 2019 population of New York City died thirty-five times. In addition to the lives saved, by the elimination of smallpox, there was also an end to the suffering, disfigurement, and blindness of those who would otherwise have been harmed by it. If you lined up all the people who have lived since 1980 because smallpox was eliminated and took one minute to greet each of them, you would spend the next 144 years meeting people who did not die of smallpox.

7 The Twentieth-century Anti-vaccine Movement

In the early twentieth century there was a lull in anti-vaccine activity. The legal parameters of vaccination became settled at the end of the nineteenth century by amendment in Britain, and a Supreme Court case in the United States. These laws allowed objectors to opt out of vaccination, but not necessarily to participate in public schools if unvaccinated. Anti-vaccine activists and public health officials had reached an uneasy detente.

Despite this, the anti-vaccination views of previous decades were still influential. In 1921 Mahatma Gandhi, the leader of the Indian independence movement and a prolific writer, published *A Guide to Health*, outlining his views on disease. Gandhi wrote that he believed that smallpox is not a contagious disease but, rather, is caused by "the blood getting impure owing to some disorder of the bowels; and the poison that accumulates in the system is expelled in the form of small-pox."[1]

On vaccination he wrote, "Vaccination is a barbarous practice, and it is one of the most fatal of all the delusions current in our time, not to be found even among the so-called savage races of the world. Its supporters are not content with its adoption by those who have no objection to it, but seek to impose it with the aid of penal laws and rigorous punishments on all people alike," and "I cannot also help feeling that vaccination is a violation of the dictates of religion and morality. The drinking of the blood of even dead animals is looked upon with horror even by habitual meat-eaters. Yet, what is vaccination but the taking in of the poisoned blood of an innocent living animal? Better far were it for God-fearing men that they should a thousand times become the victims of small-pox and even die a terrible death than that they should be guilty of such an act of sacrilege."[2]

He outlined five arguments he had against vaccination: that the preparation of vaccine involved the suffering of innocent cows; that vaccination could spread diseases other than smallpox; that the smallpox vaccine could not guarantee immunity; that vaccines were filthy; and that disease could not be cured by filth.

However, by 1930 Gandhi may have changed his mind, at least partially. After a smallpox outbreak in which he saw several children die after their parents did not have them vaccinated, in deference to Gandhi's views, he is reported to have said, "I can't sleep. These kiddies are fading away like little buds. I feel the weight of their deaths on my shoulders. I prevailed upon their parents not to get them vaccinated. Now the children are passing away. It may be, I am afraid, the result of my ignorance and obstinacy; and so I feel very unhappy," and although he himself did not believe in vaccination, he would not stand in the way of parents who wanted to have their children vaccinated.[3]

From Gandhi's perspective these views made some sense. Vaccination was a treatment being imposed by the oppressive government that he opposed. That imposition took away the bodily autonomy of the people he was fighting for. It must have seemed like just another way to control people in the most intimate possible way. The British Raj imposed vaccination without making an effort to understand the cultural context into which it was being introduced and the way the practice itself would be viewed.

In the early twentieth century, polio was reaching its peak as a recurring scourge. Parents were fearful of allowing their children to play outside in the summer, unaware of how polio was transmitted and having seen its debilitating effects. Polio could produce paralysis and death. In the 1930s two teams had worked to develop vaccines, with disastrous results. John Kolmer of Temple University had developed a vaccine through attenuation of live polio virus by passage in rhesus macaques.[4] Kolmer's vaccine was tested in ten thousand children. Jeremiah Milbank and Maurice Brodie worked on another version of the polio vaccine, this one using virus that had been inactivated by formaldehyde. This vaccine was also tested in thousands of children in the same year. Brodie's vaccine didn't produce evidence of effectiveness but did produce allergic reactions. Between the two vaccines, six children died and ten were paralyzed.

Following these tragic deaths, justified public outrage has been argued to have set back the search for a cure by two decades.[5] The anti-vivisectionist movement exaggerated the degree of human experimentation being done and framed the experiments as the testing of vaccines on orphans, though Kolmer had sought parents' permission and Brodie had tested the vaccine on himself.

Fifteen years later a series of polio epidemics made the need for a vaccine very clear. A new race began to develop the first widespread safe polio vaccine, and two approaches were used. Jonas Salk used virus grown in culture and then killed with formalin. Another form of polio vaccine, under development by Albert Sabin, used attenuated virus. This virus was grown in nonhuman cultured cells under conditions that introduced mutations. After a number of passages, the mutated virus was less effective at infecting human cells but was similar enough to wild strains of polio to still produce immunity in humans.

Salk's vaccine was developed first, in 1952, and within a few years became one of the most widely tested biologics in history with more than six hundred thousand participants. The March of Dimes[6] led a mass immunization campaign, and the incidents of polio in the United States dropped from thirty-five thousand cases in 1953 to fewer than six thousand four years later. In 1955 Sabin first presented promising results for his attenuated polio vaccine. Each vaccine type had both advantages and disadvantages. The inactivated vaccine was less long-lasting and required additional injections to provide long-term protection. The live-attenuated vaccine could be taken orally and thus protect the throat, one of the main entryways for polio into the body. However, the live-attenuated vaccine carried a small risk of causing cases of vaccine-derived polio. With the oral vaccine, the attenuated virus reproduces in the gastrointestinal tract and is shed in feces, where in poor sanitary conditions with populations that have poor vaccine coverage, it can be spread to others. Under these conditions the live virus can mutate and become more virulent as it spreads. After billions of vaccinations with the oral polio vaccine, a handful of such outbreaks have occurred, and in 2016 the oral polio vaccine was modified to make this complication less likely, and these outbreaks have been stopped by immunization of the surrounding population with more oral polio vaccine. While Salk's vaccine became the predominant form used in the United States, Sabin's attenuated virus vaccine has been used to vaccinate far more people worldwide.

In April 1955 one of the worst pharmaceutical accidents in modern history began to unfold as it became clear that more than one hundred thousand doses of polio vaccine produced by Cutter and Wyeth Laboratories had been improperly inactivated and so resulted in 250 cases of paralytic polio and 11 deaths. The reports were of paralysis only in the limb that had been injected, suggesting strongly that the vaccine had caused the infection. These incidents shook public trust in the new polio vaccine and led to the development of a permanent committee to test all lots of polio vaccine before their release to the public.[7]

The aftermath of the Cutter and Wyeth incident has continued to influence vaccine policy and opposition to the present day. Some parents began to believe that vaccination was inherently unsafe. Some medical professionals even refused to participate in the polio vaccination program due to a perceived risk of contamination. The British Medical Research Council halted trials of Salk's vaccine, and a number of European countries stopped planned immunization programs.[8] However, the Cutter and Wyeth incident also led to much stricter oversight and testing of vaccine manufacturing. Even if anti-vaccine activists today are unaware of the incident, they are likely to have been influenced by the events that followed it.

In 1974 the scientists Kulenkampff, Schwartzman, and Wilson published "Neurological Complications of Pertussis Inoculation."[9] This paper alleged that the combined diphtheria, pertussis, and tetanus vaccine, DPT, had caused encephalopathy (brain disease) in thirty-six children, including symptoms such as convulsions, spasms, screaming, vomiting, unconsciousness, or infection anywhere from zero hours to two weeks after any of four DPT injections or boosters. These patients were selected because of the severity of the alleged symptoms and a belief by the scientists that the symptoms were related to a DPT inoculation. The findings of the paper would later turn out not to be true, as sometimes happens in the scientific literature, but once published the authors could no longer control how their paper was used.

Small clinical reports of this sort are common, and the advice given in this report to look for complications following DPT inoculation was modest and even reasonable. The public reaction that followed, however, was large and revived vaccine fears that had lingered following the Cutter and Wyeth incident. The paper came out at a time when disability politics were changing and a number of policies were being enacted with the goal of improving the lives of the disabled. In 1973 the Association of Parents of Vaccine Damaged Children (APVDC) was founded by Rosemary Fox and Renee Lennon, mothers who blamed their children's brain damage on the polio vaccine and wanted to "form a society for children brain damaged by vaccination, so that from a position of strength they can put pressure on the Government for compensation."[10] In March of that year, an anonymous letter had been published in the *British Medical Journal*, proposing that Britain adopt a compensation scheme similar to those of other European nations, where anyone with a disability caused by vaccination could seek money from the government.[11] The letter provided justification in the form of an ethical argument—that if there is a small risk to the individual posed by vaccination, and vaccination benefited society as a whole, then the government should compensate those rare individuals who are unlucky and harmed.[12] Effectively this is the same argument that underlies the "vaccine court" in the United States.

Armed with a moral argument, and modeling tactics based on successful disability-advocacy groups, the APVDC sought legislation that would bring compensation from the government. The 1974 paper seemed to support their mission, so to the APVDC, the paper took on outsized importance. The APVDC decided to focus on the DPT vaccine to create doubt surrounding vaccines and was able to point to this paper as evidence. Their campaign was effective in convincing parents not to vaccinate. By 1977 vaccination rates had dropped by 50 percent and an outbreak of disease seemed likely.

Eventually the government capitulated, hoping to mollify the APVDC and allay public fears by setting up a compensation program. The result was the Vaccine Damage Payments Act of 1979. Despite this success, the APVDC took much of the blame for the 1979 pertussis epidemic that followed. Starting in 1979 and continuing into the early 1980s, an outbreak of pertussis occurred.[13] Following this outbreak, immunization rates recovered and even surpassed pre-1974 levels, reaching roughly 95 percent.

However, the effects of this campaign and the 1974 paper were felt worldwide. In 1982 "Vaccine Roulette," a television report produced by the Washington, DC–based NBC-affiliate WRC-TV, aired. The thirty-minute program spent eleven minutes showing images of disabled children and less than two minutes on a girl with whooping cough.[14] The program prompted thousands of worried calls to physicians and officials. In 1986 the book *DPT: A Shot in the Dark* argued that pertussis vaccination was dangerous. Despite the public concerns these raised, immunization rates remained high in the United States, as they did in Poland, Hungary, and the former East Germany.

In Sweden DPT vaccination rates dropped from 90 percent in 1974 to 12 percent in 1979, and pertussis outbreaks followed in 1983 and 1985.[15] Between 1981 and 1983, 4 percent of patients hospitalized for pertussis developed neurological complications, 14 percent of whom developed pneumonia, and three children died. In Japan a movement arose against pertussis vaccination, and the Ministry of Health and Welfare eliminated whole-cell pertussis vaccination. Rates of vaccination fell from 80 percent in 1974 to 10 percent in 1976. Here again an outbreak followed, resulting in forty-one deaths before a new vaccine was introduced. In the Russian Federation several pediatricians led a campaign against pertussis vaccination, which led in turn to a drop in confidence and epidemics. In Ireland vaccination dropped to 30 percent in 1976, and epidemics occurred in 1985 and 1989. In Australia the same story: a drop in confidence, followed by medical providers ceasing recommendation, followed by an outbreak of pertussis.

A pattern emerged from the way these countries had reacted to suggestions of a link between pertussis vaccination and neurological disorders. In countries where anti-vaccine rhetoric had taken hold but public health officials maintained strong disease surveillance, took measures to reassure the public, and maintained strong immunization programs, pertussis did not return. In countries where doubts took hold and public health officials capitulated by moving away from pertussis vaccination, vaccination rates dropped and outbreaks occurred. The outbreaks ceased once immunization resumed. This conclusion is compatible with research showing that the motivations of governments and individuals differ when it comes to immunization decisions. Governments are primarily concerned with costs, whereas individuals are primarily concerned with perceived risks. Collectively vaccination protects nonvaccinated individuals through herd immunity as well. Absent collective motivations, individuals would choose to vaccinate at lower rates.[16]

In the United States, the DPT scare resulted in a series of lawsuits filed against the three manufacturers of the DPT vaccine. Wyeth Laboratories stopped manufacturing the vaccine because

of their low profitability and the risk of litigation.[17] By 1984 Con-
naught Laboratories, the second of the three major manufacturers of the vaccine, had halted production, citing risk of lawsuits.
These stoppages led to a shortage of pertussis vaccine.[18] The
number of lawsuits filed related to the DPT vaccine rose from 2
suits in 1978 to more than 250 suits in 1986, the latter seeking
a total of $3.162 billion.[19] Several large payouts were awarded,
and several settlements were reached. Where doubt had been
created, lawyers swarmed, demanding large payouts for their clients and themselves. The shortage created by these legal actions
put DPT vaccination rates at risk of dropping, and public health
officials became concerned that an outbreak might occur.

The National Childhood Vaccine Injury Act (NCVIA) of 1986
was the US Congress's response to this risk to vaccine availability. The act's intent was both to create a system for monitoring
possible unknown reactions from vaccines and to allow patients
who met certain criteria to receive compensation without
threatening the supply of vaccines necessary to maintain public health. The act recognized that the private manufacture of
vaccines, which were necessary for public health, required legal
protections. When manufacture is unprofitable, corporations
lose interest.

One of the more notable outcomes of this act was the establishment of the National Vaccine Injury Compensation Program
(VICP) in 1988 to compensate those whose children were injured
by routine childhood vaccinations. Although the concerns
about the DTP vaccine turned out to be unfounded, occasionally
adverse reactions do occur with some vaccines. The VICP provides a list of such reactions, and patients who experience these
events within a specified time frame may ask for compensation.
The program now compensates medical and legal costs, provides

up to $250,000 for pain and suffering, and offers a death benefit
of $250,000. Legal fees may be covered, even if a claim is not
accepted.[20]

Occasionally the existence of the "vaccine court," or compensation to those seeking it through the VICP, is used by anti-
vaccine activists to suggest that there is broad recognition that
vaccines are, in fact, genuinely dangerous. However, legal standards of evidence are not the same as scientific standards of
evidence. Legal judgments don't determine scientific truth. The
VICP has a standard of evidence lower than that used in criminal
trials or scientific research. The VICP will compensate based on
a "preponderance of evidence"—a term that means that the person evaluating the evidence for a claim believes there is a more
than a 50 percent probability that a proposition is true.[21]

In 2005 *Althen v. Secretary of Health and Human Services*[22] found
that in an individual case where the court had required "confirmation of medical plausibility from the medical community and
literature," the NCVIA did not require "objective confirmation,"
in its standard of evidence, only medical records or medical
opinion. Effectively, the ruling in this case lowered the standard
of evidence such that biological plausibility and scientific evidence were irrelevant to legal determinations for compensation
for vaccine injury.

Starting in 2008, this lowered standard of evidence came into
play in several cases in subsequent years, allowing compensation for a variety of ailments with no biologically plausible link
to vaccination, such as chronic fatigue syndrome, fibromyal-
gia, and multiple sclerosis.[23] One well-publicized case was that
of Hannah Poling,[24] who at nineteen months received vaccines
for diphtheria, tetanus, acellular pertussis, Hib, MMR, varicella,
and polio. Several months later she developed symptoms of a

developmental delay and was diagnosed with encephalopathy caused by a mitochondrial-enzyme deficit. The Polings won compensation through the VICP, despite an absence of biological plausibility, or scientific evidence of causation. They held a press conference announcing the legal ruling, and the Centers for Disease Control and Prevention (CDC) responded, pointing out that the ruling was not proof of a link between vaccines and autism. Nevertheless, this case has been used by anti-vaccine activists to suggest that a link between vaccinations and autism has been proven in a court of law.

Legal rulings have no bearing on scientific and medical truth. Like scientists, legal professionals are interested in finding the truth (well, at least sometimes). However, the means that the legal profession uses to arrive at decisions are different from those used in science. In a legal ruling, a decision must be reached. In scientific inquiry, the starting point of every investigation, "I don't know," is the default epistemological standpoint, and most common endpoint for an investigation. There are not specific rules that scientists must follow to the letter while evaluating evidence; however, there are heuristics and scientific virtues that scientists follow and apply when conducting, evaluating, and peer reviewing evidence. Results published in the scientific literature are not considered to be final but may at any time be reconsidered in the light of additional evidence, conflicting experiments, or new discoveries. Only rarely does a scientific proposition rise to the point where it is considered to be a "theory," which is accepted to be true pending further evidence, or a new model that better explains existing data. Legal rulings by the VICP do not determine scientific truth; rather, they determine if a case presented meets the standards set out in law. These standards are often flawed and partial. So the ruling that Dorothy Poling was entitled to compensation under the VICP was a ruling that she met the legal requirements set forth in the law to receive compensation; this ruling did not bear on the scientific question.

The NCVIA also led to the establishment of the Vaccine Adverse Event Reporting System (VAERS). This system allows health-care providers and individuals to report adverse events following vaccination so that the CDC and the Food and Drug Administration (FDA) can detect unknown adverse reactions to vaccines, identify factors that might cause some patients to be at risk for reactions, identify safety issues, and identify bad batches or clusters of vaccines should they occur. VAERS requires health-care providers to report certain events—such as shoulder injuries related to the administration of the vaccine, fainting, and death—within a specified time window following vaccination.

Those who are not health-care workers may also report to VAERs, and there is no requirement that events reported to VAERS be factually associated with vaccination. This has been exploited. Following the discredited 1998 *Lancet* article attempting to draw a link between the MMR vaccine and autism, the number of reports of autism through VAERS spiked.[25] Those making those reports disproportionately associated the vaccine with autism, many citing personal websites as sources of information. A 2006 study showed that over time, the number of VAERS reports related to litigation was increasing and that a disproportionate fraction of these reports were filed by lawyers seeking litigation.[26] To demonstrate that associations made by using this data were of dubious value, James Laidler submitted a VAERS report claiming that following influenza vaccination, he had turned into the comics character the Hulk.[27] He was asked to withdraw the report and did. Despite these limitations, VAERS is a useful tool for legitimate researchers hoping to identify possible patterns of adverse events, so long as its potential limitations are understood and proper statistical methods are used.

The NCVIA also established the National Vaccine Program Office within the Department of Health and Human Services.[28] This office is responsible for coordinating between the multiple federal agencies and offices that play a role in vaccine safety, distribution, and development, as well as in staffing the National Vaccine Advisory Committee.

The NCVIA required that Vaccine Information Statements be provided by health-care providers alongside certain immunizations. These statements are developed by the CDC and contain information about the vaccine being administered, the disease being prevented, and the people who may have contraindications against vaccination. For example, the 2018 flu vaccine is contraindicated for patients with severe allergies because the production method for flu vaccine often uses eggs, which may cause allergic reactions.[29] These statements also include information about possible risks associated with the vaccine and what to do in case of an adverse reaction. Despite reporting requirements, time-limited health-care providers may not have the opportunity to provide every patient with a Vaccine Information Statement.[30]

8 Autism

Starting in the late 1990s, many of the claims made by anti-vaccine activists have been related to autism. To understand what's being discussed, it is helpful to know what autism actually is, what we know about its origins, and what we know about its treatment. Following this, we can discuss those claims in more detail.

A modern understanding recognizes autism spectrum disorder (ASD) as a broad range of neurodevelopmental disorders sharing features of repetitive behavior and difficulty both in social situations and with communication.[1] Currently 1 to 2 percent of children are diagnosed as being somewhere on the autism spectrum. In the past, the number of children diagnosed was lower. The change is mostly likely due to an improved definition and a better understanding of autism; greater access to resources for parents of autistic children, leading more to seek diagnosis; and wider access to medical care. Although no one was diagnosed with autism in the 1750s, autistic people were born at the time; there simply was no appropriate label.

The first description of autism (and the coining of the term) occurred in 1943 in "Autistic Disturbances of Affective Contact," a paper by the psychiatrist and physician Leo Kanner.[2] Kanner noted that the syndrome presented was probably more common than indicated by the small number of cases he had assembled and that several of the children he had studied had been introduced to him as "idiots or imbeciles." Since the publication of that paper, the definition of autism has expanded to include a wider breadth of behaviors and symptoms, and it is now recognized as a spectrum that can range from severe impairments to relatively minor differences in social behavior.

Part of the difficulty in defining autism comes from applying a single label to a large set of behaviors and people. It's likely that there are multiple underlying factors that can lead to the development of autistic behavior. One of the factors we want to understand about traits is the degree to which a given trait develops due to mutable environmental factors, compared to genetic or epigenetic factors that are passed down from parent to child.

When scientists want to understand the degree to which a trait is inherited, they develop a statistic called the heritability index, which indicates what fraction of the variation in a trait in a population can be explained by inheritance. As an example, the trait "stubbornness" might have a heritability index of 0.7. That does not mean that 70 percent of a person's stubbornness is caused by genes and 30 percent by environment. Rather, it means that the variation in the trait is 70 percent explained by the presence of that trait in that person's parents. In a situation where the environment changes and makes more variation in stubbornness occur, the heritability of stubbornness would increase. Some traits may be heritable, but not strictly through genetics. For example, the heritability index suggests that college education can be inherited. That does not mean that education is a genetic trait, but rather that social and environmental factors, as well, can be passed from parent to child.

The heritability index for autism is consistently measured at about 0.9. If an identical twin has autism, there is roughly a 64 percent chance that its twin also has autism, while fraternal twins, who do not share identical DNA, are only 9 percent likely to have autism if their twins have autism,[3] while their nontwin siblings have only a 3 percent chance of having autism. In about 40 percent of cases, studying the genetics of an individual with autism can point to an underlying genetic cause, such as a chromosomal abnormality such as fragile X syndrome,[4] or polymorphism that has been associated with ASD. Altogether these data strongly indicate that autism is largely controlled by inherited biological factors, including genetics.[5] In 2019 the largest and most statistically powerful study to date, which included more than two million participants, found that ASD was about 80 percent heritable.[6]

Why hasn't a single autism gene been found? Some traits, such as height, are so-called polygenic traits. This means that in humans, the variation in more than one gene can lead to the final height of an individual. There are not just tall and short humans, there is a spectrum of heights centered around a mean, or an average height, with most individuals being close to average and fewer individuals being far taller or far shorter than average. Some genetic factors, such as the presence of a Y chromosome, have a large influence on height, while other genetic factors have smaller contributions. Although a person with a Y chromosome and an X chromosome is, on average, likely to be taller than a person with two X chromosomes, there are many examples of those with Y and X chromosomes who are shorter than others with two X chromosomes. So, except in rare cases, it is not possible to know the precise combination of genetic variations that a person has based solely on knowing that person's height.[7] Likewise there is not a single gene that causes autism, and it is not possible to predict someone's genes just from the presence of autistic behaviors.

The complex set of behavioral traits to which we assign the term *autism spectrum disorder* has a complex set of genes that contribute to the final observed trait. We only know some of them, but work is ongoing to discover the others. Most likely there is a contribution from the variability of hundreds of genes.[8] The goals of this work are to discover new means of improving the quality of life for people on the autism spectrum, to offer earlier diagnosis, to provide improved educational resources, and to develop an understanding of the genes that influence the development of ASD so that potential parents might be provided better genetic counseling. Because the diagnosis of autism is based on behavior and because behavior can have many causes, we will never have a single cause that explains all cases.

The earliest detectable signs of ASD appear between the ages of two and six months, when attention to eyes declines in infants.[9] By two years of age, eye contact can be significantly impaired in children with ASD.[10] ASD is usually diagnosed in the first thirty-six months of life, although many are now diagnosed as adults. Boys are four- or three-to-one more likely than girls to be diagnosed with ASD,[11] although it's likely that girls are underdiagnosed, and studies have been highly variable in their results. The symptoms of ASD can include displaying little eye contact, delays in speech and language, difficulty with changes to environment, sensitivity to certain sensory stimuli such as smells or sounds, repetitive behaviors, and narrowed interests.

In the late 1990s, even less was known about the origins of autism than is now, people were eager to fill those gaps. Many of the anti-vaccine claims that have developed in the last two decades have referenced fears related to the development of autism in children. These claims have followed roughly two parallel tracks, which have often become conflated. The first centers around a scientific paper that claimed the combined MMR vaccine used in England resulted in a kind of "regressive autism." The second centers around the idea that thimerosal, a preservative that was used in vaccines starting in the 1930s, and largely ending in the 2000s was causing autism symptoms through a kind of heavy-metal poisoning. Both of these claims have since proven to be false.

9   The Anti-vaccine Movement, 1998–Present

Falsehood flies, and truth comes limping after, so that when men come to be undeceived, it is too late; the jest is over and the tale hath had its effect: like a man, who hath thought of a good repartee when the discourse is changed, or the company parted; or like a physician, who hath found out an infallible medicine, after the patient is dead.
—Jonathan Swift, 1710

If a single event can be said to be the trigger for the modern anti-vaccine movement, it is the publication in 1998 of "Ileal-Lymphoid-Nodular Hyperplasia, Non-specific Colitis, and Pervasive Developmental Disorder in Children," a research journal article in the *Lancet*. The primary author of this study was Andrew Wakefield. The paper claimed that there was a link between the MMR vaccine offered in England at that time and the development of a new kind of autistic regression, where otherwise healthy children started to regress in development. Later investigation showed that other scientists were unable to replicate Wakefield's results, and the investigative journalist Brian Deer showed that the paper was a significant case of scientific fraud. The paper was retracted in 2010.[1] Following this retraction Wakefield was eventually investigated and lost his license to practice medicine. He then traveled to the United States, where he has since started a variety of ventures that have taken advantage of his status as a martyr to the anti-vaccine movement. Despite these events, the media coverage of the paper played a pivotal role in setting off a major vaccine scare and a belief in a vaccine-autism link that lingers to this day.

The paper reported the cases of twelve children who had developed normally until they began losing skills and language, and developed diarrhea and abdominal pain.[2] A series of assessments were performed on the children. They were tested for abnormal neurological conditions, using techniques such as MRI and EEG, and their guts were examined endoscopically and by biopsy of the mucosa. They were also tested for coeliac disease and infections with bacteria, such as salmonella. Their urinary methylmalonic-acid levels were observed to be high, an indicator of having a vitamin B_{12} deficiency. Endoscopic images of their gastrointestinal tracts showed early indicators of Crohn's disease, as well as follicular hyperplasia, which can be symptomatic of a number of disorders. The children's histories also showed that their parent's recalled vaccinating them with the MMR vaccine just before the onset of their symptoms.

The *Lancet* paper concludes by speculating as to possible causes for the reported medical findings. One hypothesis for the cause of autism-like symptoms was an excess of opioids caused by the breakdown of certain dietary proteins into peptides, which are then absorbed in excess and interact with the nervous system. The paper drew a link between the MMR vaccine and such symptoms, noting that the first symptoms of autism appear within a few weeks of vaccination, but came short of specifying a causative relationship.

Although the *Lancet* published this article, in the same issue, they published a critical commentary.[3] The commentary acknowledged that no vaccine is perfectly safe and continued on to address the specific points made in the paper. Because vaccines are administered to many millions of people, an adverse event that occurs in even one-tenth of 1 percent of recipients would be unacceptable. Yet the mechanisms that were in place to discover and identify those events had not identified any adverse event linked to the development of autism. The commentary pointed out that in order to infer a causative relationship between vaccination and an adverse event, questions of adverse events must be addressed in a very specific way.

Just two weeks before, the *British Medical Journal* had published an editorial, reviewing how adverse media could negatively impact vaccine coverage and noting that earlier reports linking MMR to inflammatory bowel disease had not stood up to scientific inquiry, but had already had negative effects. The editorial referenced a 1993 Danish television station that had aired anti-vaccination programming, leading to the lowest coverage rate yet.[4] These papers in the *BMJ* and *Lancet* suggest that a number of people were aware of the impending publication of the *Lancet* paper and were unhappy with the editorial decision.

Although a report like the one that the *Lancet* had published could potentially point in new directions for research, or provide such prior probability to look for a connection in data between vaccination and bowel disease, it did not on its own do the kind of large statistical test that would be necessary to say such an effect really existed in the population. Indeed, although the number of measles cases reported had declined significantly due to the widespread vaccination of millions of children, among those many millions, no reports had been recorded of bowel disease or behavioral problems developing post-vaccination.

The symptoms reported in the *Lancet* article were not unique or particularly rare, and they had existed before the introduction of the MMR vaccine. One explanation for the parents in the study associating the onset of symptoms with MMR vaccination is recall bias. Recall bias occurs when asking someone to retrospectively report events; it makes it difficult for people to accurately recall when the onset of symptoms began.[5] Asking someone "When did the symptoms start?" will always lead to less accurate answers than will asking them to record symptoms as they appear.

Additionally, the proposed mechanism of association: vaccination causing irritable bowel syndrome that then caused autism did not match the order of events in the reported cases. The patients had noticed the development of behavioral symptoms before that of bowel symptoms. The *Lancet* commentary pointed out that many developmental disorders appear in the first years of life, which is the same time period when most vaccinations occur. Assuming a causative effect simply from proximity in time invites making false associations.

> Vaccine-safety concerns such as that reported by Wakefield and colleagues may snowball into societal tragedies when the media and the public confuse association with causality and shun immunisation.[6]

In the same issue, the *Lancet* published a research letter examining samples from patients with Crohn's disease and ulcerative colitis, forms of inflammatory bowel disease. If measles was the cause of inflammation in these diseases, it would be expected that genetic material from measles could be detected in these samples. No such association was shown.[7]

To scientists reading this issue of the *Lancet*, the inclusion of this commentary and this research letter sent a clear message. Although the journal had gone ahead with the publication of the early report suggesting a link between the development of autism and vaccination, the editors were skeptical of the conclusions. Indeed, three meetings were held to determine if the journal should go ahead with publishing the study. As written, the study appeared to have been conducted properly, and the appropriate methods and protocols appeared to have been followed. The results, if true, were important enough to warrant publication. The usual tests for publication are validity of the methods used and importance to the field.

However, as the commentary and research letter showed, the results seemed incongruous with respect to the existing literature, and even potentially dangerous. The editors were aware of the vaccine fears that had been rekindled in the 1970s by the report in the *British Medical Journal* suggesting a link between the DPT and neurological deficits in thirty-six children,[8] as they had published a history of it the previous month, in January 1998,[9] detailing how the airing of "Vaccine Roulette" had led to public health concerns in the United States and eventually to worldwide pertussis outbreaks.

The publication of this history just before that of the 1998 *Lancet* paper was, if not deliberate, then eerily prescient. The editors faced a hard choice but decided to go ahead with publication, but not to include the paper in their normal press release. Although the journal chose not to publicize the paper, the Royal Free Hospital, Wakefield's employer, did choose to directly address the media in a press conference to be held before the paper's publication. Five doctors, each with different views on the paper, were called into a panel. All five rehearsed and agreed that until further research could be done, MMR vaccinations should continue. This agreement fell apart during the conference, with Andrew Wakefield advocating individual vaccines in annual intervals and others disagreeing vehemently.[10] Stating that MMR was dangerous far exceeded what even Wakefield's paper concluded. Although Wakefield suggested that the combined MMR vaccine was dangerous and that individual vaccines would be safer, none were available on the market at that time, an absence that effectively told parents not to vaccinate.

> One more case of this is too many.... It's a moral issue for me and I can't support the continued use of these three vaccines given in combination until this issue has been resolved.[11]

The damage had been done. In the press the next day, alarming headlines suggested that the *Lancet* article should provoke immediate action. The front page of the *Guardian* reported, "Alert over Child Jabs." In the following years, MMR immunization fell from 91.5 percent of children by the age of two to a low of only 79 percent in 2004.[12] Alarm about a claimed link between vaccinations and autism took on a life of its own in subsequent years. It led to a series of congressional hearings covered on widely watched news programs,[13] decreases in vaccination rates, and a number of sick children. Some of this anti-vaccine panic may have arisen even in the absence of this paper, but Wakefield and others who followed provided a scientific veneer to holding anti-vaccine beliefs, creating an alternate narrative for those who wanted to believe that a conspiracy of ill-behaved humans was responsible for autism, rather than the intentionless actions of many genes interacting with unpredictable elements in the environment.

Over the course of several years, it became clear that the *Lancet* article had been produced under irregular circumstances. In

2004 the investigative journalist Brian Deer published a piece in the *Sunday Times* revealing that in August 1996 Wakefield had secured up to £55,000 (roughly $210,000 today) to investigate a possible link between MMR and autism in ten children by the Legal Aid Board. A month later he sent a letter to the government's chief medical officer urging against the MMR vaccine. Four to five of the children in the study published in the *Lancet* were covered in Wakefield's contract to look for a link between autism and MMR.

Scientific journals provide an opportunity to declare conflicts of interest, which are often minor. Doing occasional consulting work for a company whose drug is tested in a study is one such conflict that may be reported and is considered by editors when deciding to accept or reject an article. Wakefield did not declare his conflict—that he had been paid, in effect, to draw a link between the MMR vaccine and autism in order to justify legal proceedings. This clear conflict of interest was not disclosed to the public or to coauthors of the manuscript.[14] The editor who had approved the article stated that had he known about the conflict, he would not have approved publication.

Wakefield admitted that children had been included in the study because he had been paid to help them make a legal case. Following Deer's investigative journalism, the Royal Free Hospital, University College medical school, and the Royal Free Hampstead NHS Trust released a statement: had they known about the conflict of interest, they would have advised reporting it.[15] Ten of the paper's twelve authors later issued a "Retraction of an Interpretation" statement, wherein they stated, "We wish to make it clear that in this paper no causal link was established between MMR vaccine and autism as the data were insufficient."[16] Wakefield filed a libel suit against Deer, which was soon dropped.

A solicitor, Richard Barr, had been pursuing cases related to injuries that parents believed were caused by vaccination. Barr had used an organization called Justice, Awareness, and Basic Support (JABS)[17] to approach and pay Wakefield to research a proposed link between MMR and autism. Over time Wakefield would be paid £435,643 (just above $1 million today adjusted for inflation) plus expenses.[18] JABS members were involved in a lawsuit against the three companies that manufactured the MMR vaccine.[19] Wakefield had already tried to show a link between MMR and intestinal inflammation, so it made sense to approach him to look for a link between MMR and another disorder.

Although the journalistic world had been quick to respond to the 1998 paper by promoting and amplifying its findings, the scientific world responded more slowly and measuredly. In March 1998 the *Lancet* published a rebuttal to the Wakefield paper,[20] pointing out that developmental delays are noticed slowly over time, not immediately or all at once; that the selection of patients was not blinded; that the study did not have controls;[21] that researchers were not blinded;[22] and that if symptoms were first observed soon after vaccination, this was not enough to make an inference that vaccination was the *cause* of symptoms.

The same month, the *British Medical Journal* published an editorial with similar conclusions.[23] Although hundreds of thousands of children were vaccinated annually, there was no epidemiological reason to associate MMR with autism. The World Health Organization had reviewed the biological and epidemiological plausibility of such an association,[24] finding that there was little evidence to implicate measles as a cause of inflammatory bowel disease and that "current scientific data do not permit a causal link to be drawn between the measles virus and [chronic inflammatory bowel disease]." Indeed, a number of studies attempted to look at the question of whether the measles virus used in MMR vaccination was a causative factor in inflammatory bowel disease.[25] These had failed to confirm this hypothesis.[26]

In June 1999 the *Lancet* published a study of 498 cases of autism.[27] Notably the presence of autism as diagnosed by the International Classification of Diseases was used as a criterion for inclusion in the study, and not whether a participant's parents had paid the investigators to help build a legal case. The investigators found that there was no association between the time of vaccination and the onset of symptoms of autism, a finding that dealt a blow to Wakefield's MMR-vaccination hypothesis.

Studies continued to look for the proposed link. Compared to nonregressing children, autistic children who appeared to have regressed did not have symptoms appear at a different time, and inflammatory bowel disease did not appear to be more frequent in these children.[28] The diagnosis of autism increased from 1988 to 1999, by seven times, but the vaccination rate had remained relatively stable at about 95 percent.[29]

A retrospective study of over 500,000 children found no increased risk of developing autism symptoms in the months following vaccination and no link between children with autism and hospitalizations for inflammatory bowel disease.[30] Incidence of bowel symptoms and incidence of developmental regression did not change from before the time that the MMR vaccine was introduced to after.[31] A case-control study of hundreds of autistic and non-autistic children calculated the odds ratio that increasing exposure to vaccine components increased the risk of autism. An odds ratio = 1 indicates that exposure does not influence the odds of the outcome. An odds ratio > 1 indicates that exposure is associated with a higher risk of outcome, and an odds ratio < 1 indicates that exposure is associated with a lower risk of outcome.[32] The odds ratio was 0.999 for exposure up to three months, 0.999 for exposure up to seven months, and 0.999 for exposure up to two years,[33] indicating that there was no relationship between vaccine exposure and diagnosis with autism. A 2014 meta-analysis studied the combined outcomes of available high-quality studies and found no relationship between vaccination and autism, vaccination and autism spectrum disorder, autism and MMR, autism and thimerosal, and autism and mercury.[34]

Dozens of studies have been conducted looking for a link between MMR and autism, with multiple methodologies employed and many more participants than Wakefield's study, and all have reached the same conclusion: there is no link between the MMR vaccine and the development of autism, the development of inflammatory bowel disease, or the development of a new subtype of autism characterized by developmental regression.

The quantity and quality of this scientific body of work is impossible to ignore in an honest inquiry conducted by someone with scientific training. Did the media cover the findings of the scientists studying these questions as breathlessly and with as much excitement as it did Wakefield's? It did not. In 2002 the BBC aired an episode of *Panorama* titled "How Safe Is MMR?" The *Sun* and the *Daily Mail* argued for individual vaccines for measles, mumps, and rubella,[35] a practice that can increase the period during which children are vulnerable to infection. Many news outlets attempted to provide "balance" when discussing vaccination;[36] however, although balance is a journalistic virtue when reporting on disputes, adding balance to a scientific question often elevates an extreme minority position, such as Wakefield's, to a disproportionate position of false equivalence. This is frequently called false balance.

Celebrities began to weigh in. Jenny McCarthy first declared her son to be a "crystal child," in 2006, then later, autistic. It is unclear whether her son was ever medically diagnosed with autism. She appeared on *The Oprah Winfrey Show*, *Larry King Live*, and *Frontline* claiming that vaccines can cause autism. In 2008 she was awarded the James Randi Educational Foundation's Pigasus Award[37] for contributions to pseudoscience. Jenna Elfman appeared at a rally against California's law (SB-277) tightening rules on vaccine exemptions, on the basis that it infringed on parental rights. Jim Carrey wrote an editorial for the *Huffington Post*, suggesting a link between vaccines and autism.[38] Alicia Silverstone wrote a parenting book that opposed giving childhood vaccinations (as well as using diapers and eating meat and dairy while pregnant).[39] Kirstie Alley tweeted against SB-277, and a variety of other celebrities issued anti-vaccine tweets, including Selma Blair, game show host and former real estate developer Donald Trump, Erin Brockovich, and Bill Maher.[40]

Shortly after McCarthy went on a press tour to promote her book, ABC aired the first episode of *Eli Stone*, featuring a corporate lawyer who suffers from hallucinations and decides to "fight for the little guy," by taking on a pharmaceutical company on behalf of a parent who believes a fictionalized version of the vaccine-preservative thimerosal had caused her child's autism.[41] The episode was protested by a number of professional groups, including the American Academy of Pediatrics; however, it was aired regardless with a warning that the company portrayed was fictional.[42]

Of course, celebrities often gain their fame for reasons other than their ability to evaluate and interpret evidence. Skills at acting, playing sports, or making media appearances are not the same as such skills as evaluating scientific evidence and making choices based on the best available data. Having platforms able to interest in knowing that the change in temperature of the river water is killing fish and causing other environmental damage, so the journalist works diligently to ascertain what happened without reporting the corporation's statement that the waste water is safe, absent their own fact-checking and interpretation.

Likewise, when interviewing scientists and institutional leaders, journalists see scientists, as well as business leaders and politicians, as parties with individual interests, as potentially biased holders of power. Scientists have their own set of social functions and intellectual virtues. Science develops new and life-saving technologies, new weapons, and new tools. It helps us to understand the world we live in; the living things that occupy it; our own behavior; and our biological, physical and chemical origins.

Journalists also work on a deadline. Although scientists are motivated to publish, the pace of scientific research often rewards patience and getting things right. A single scientific publication might represent several years' worth of work and may take several rounds of peer review, new experiments, and revision before it is accepted into a reputable journal. Although desiring to only present factual information, a journalist with a deadline to deliver a story before the publication of a newspaper or the airing of television program may simply not have enough time to "get it right" because they interviewed the wrong people, missed important features, or were not able to follow up on sources. Long-form investigative journalism, such as Deer's investigation of Wakefield's conflicts of interest, can slowly fill these gaps.

Science often falls for the so-called file-drawer effect, wherein negative results are unreported and have a harder time getting published.[44] This causes problems in its own right, increasing the risk of reported false positives and resulting in studies repeated by various groups because the negative results of prior groups aren't available. News media tend to emphasize negative stories or use negative frames when reporting stories.[45] Humans are also apt to see studies that find health risks as more trustworthy than those that show low or no risk.[46] As a result, news is biased toward reporting negative stories, those that portray institutions or individuals as villains, and those that present opportunities for the media to serve its role as a watchdog. This can in turn lead to greater availability of information suggesting risk, which may in turn increase a person's perception of the likelihood of a dangerous event taking place.[47] Since the news is, by definition, new, stories that upend the status quo will naturally be more appealing to report than those that reinforce it.

Science journalism can't be said to be uniformly bad. The quality of scientific news falls on a spectrum.[48] Some venues provide very accurate coverage that is novel and reflects the scientific consensus. Other outlets, often with wider reach, spread misinformation.

One recent philosophical approach to epistemology (the study of knowledge) may help to bridge the divide between science and the news media. Virtue epistemology frames the pursuit of knowledge not by a codified set of fixed techniques and mechanisms but by drawing an analogy to moral virtues. A scientist holds such epistemic virtues as doing hypothesis-driven research, keeping meticulous notes, and maintaining clean glassware. A journalist may hold such virtues as balance, following up on sources, and cross validation of results. By understanding the journalistic virtues, and how journalists conceive of their role in society, scientists may be better able to navigate situations where they must interact with journalists in order to tell scientific stories and spread accurate public health information.

Journalists should be aware that scientific ways of knowing fall outside of the approaches they're used to employing for getting to the truth. In science, those stories that upend the status quo are often the least interesting because they're most likely to be false. In science, individual opinions hold little weight, and individual interviews can be next to useless for determining facts. Rarely do issues have "two sides" of equal scientific merit that deserve equal representation. Credentials alone mean little. Those representing themselves as scientists or physicians may well have doctorates, but they may also be speaking well outside their areas of expertise. The story of the little guy going up against an evil corporation may make for a compelling (and well-worn) narrative, but often the little guy is working with bad science. Scientists often speak very carefully using precise and qualified language—for the reason that care must be taken to accurately portray their views. Patronizing "simplification" of scientists' communication often simply leads to confusion as statements that made sense in context become weaker, more easily assailable, or flat wrong.

Brian Deer continued to investigate Wakefield's paper. He tracked down parents of children involved in the study who provided medical records contradicting what had been reported.[49] The General Medical Council (GMC) spent 217 days evaluating the Wakefield case (its longest-ever disciplinary hearing) and in January 2010 found Wakefield to have committed misconduct related to his paper.[50] Young children had undergone invasive procedures such as endoscopies and lumbar puncture; however, these procedures had not been reviewed by the appropriate ethics panel. In February 2010 the *Lancet* retracted the 1998 paper. In March 2010 the GMC removed Wakefield from the medical register.

Moreover, many of the specific claims made in the paper began to fall apart. Many of the children documented in the paper had been diagnosed not with regressive autism but with Asperger's syndrome, or with nothing at all. Some of the children, who had been believed to be "previously normal," had previously documented developmental delays or abnormalities. Deer showed that all the children in the study in some way had their case histories altered or misrepresented to fit the paper's narrative.

In another report, Deer revealed that Wakefield had filed a patent in 1995 for a method of detecting Crohn's disease from measles virus in "bowel tissue, bowel products, or body fluids."[51] The application had suggested that the service could be the basis for a profitable company. Richard Barr, the lawyer who had paid Wakefield, directly stated that he had paid for the *Lancet* research. After the press conference, Wakefield held a meeting with a venture capitalist about launching "Immunospecifics Bio-technologies Ltd." The company was to market a stand-alone measles vaccine. In 2001 Wakefield was presented with a letter expressing concerns that the business he was launching had a business plan based on yet-undemonstrated research and that this caused a conflict of interest with his work at the Royal Free Hospital. An offer was made to Wakefield to replicate the results of his *Lancet* study with more children, but he failed to do so. He was paid severance and lost his job at the hospital.

Wakefield has publicly denied any wrongdoing and refused to retract his initial paper. An interview for this book was requested through his assistant; however, Wakefield never responded. In various interviews he has asserted a conspiracy as the cause of negative interpretations of his work. Deer's interpretation, and the interpretation of most scientists, was that Wakefield had

performed scientific misconduct.[52] He had received payment
to produce plausibility in the scientific literature to help a lawsuit move forward and to market his own alternative measles
vaccine. He hid this when conducting the study, violated ethics rules in examining the children, and misrepresented their
patient histories and diagnoses. This case of research misconduct
also throws his other publications into question.

In the years after Wakefield's separation from the Royal Free
Hospital, he eventually moved to the United States. In 2004, in
Austin, Texas, he helped found the Thoughtful House Center for
Children, where he was said to be in charge of research[53] and was
executive director, earning about $250,000 a year.[54] He eventu-
ally resigned in 2010, around the time of his GMC hearings. In
2011 the institution's name was changed to the Johnson Center for Child Health and Development. Wakefield then started
a charity, the Strategic Autism Initiative (SAI). As of 2012 about
58 percent of the money SAI had taken in went to salaries, with
the majority going to Wakefield.[55] In 2012 more was spent on
salaries than was taken in. By 2013 SAI took in only $50,498
and ran a deficit of $97,514 according to tax forms. Also in 2010
Wakefield registered a company called the Autism File Global,
amended in 2011 to the Autism Media Channel.

In 2010 Wakefield gave a talk to Somali-Americans in Minnesota incorrectly claiming that autism does not exist in Soma-
lia.[56] In 2017 this community would be the center of the largest
measles outbreak in Minnesota in recent memory.

In 2013, representing the Autism Media Channel, Wakefield
pitched a "reality" television program about an "Autism Team"
that diagnoses children with "autism-associated enterocolitis"
and then cures the children.[57] *Autism-associated enterocolitis* is a
term invented by Wakefield and not a recognized disease. The

10   Vaxxed

Vaxxed is a film that fails to be an objective presentation of facts, if it ever strived to be that. It starts with a conclusion held to be true by its principals and then works backward to build a story that, through ideological cherry picking, seems to support that conclusion.

In 2009 the authors of the article "Denialism: What Is It, and How Should Scientists Respond?" sought to define *science denial* as constituted by five features that are shared in part or in total by denial.[1] The first is relying on conspiracy theories to explain a scientific consensus. The second is using fake experts—people who pretend to have specific expertise but whose views go against established knowledge; together with this is attempting to discredit established experts. The third is cherry-picking data, or selecting only isolated papers that go against the dominant consensus. The fourth is demanding that science deliver impossible results, by being always perfect, or testing impossible questions. The fifth is using faulty logic. *Vaxxed* meets all of these criteria.

Vaxxed primarily focuses on a conspiracy theory centering on what it calls a fraud conducted by the CDC in interpreting data in a study that the film's authors believe showed a link between childhood MMR vaccination and the onset of symptoms in

African American boys. This is an example of both cherry-picking and relying on conspiracy theories.

The 2004 study used a case-control design to examine 624 children with autism in Atlanta-area schools matched to 1,824 nonautistic children in Atlanta-area schools.[2] Case-control studies are good at looking for causes of rare diseases because rather than selecting a large population and hoping to get enough people with the disease, they identify the people with the disease and then include them in the study.

In the 2004 study, forms that were required for children to enter school were used to establish times of vaccination. Birth certificates were used to determine "maternal and birth factors." The study found that similar numbers of autistic and nonautistic children had been vaccinated with MMR between twelve and seventeen months of age (70.5 percent and 67.5 percent, respectively), and slightly more children with autism had been vaccinated before thirty-six months of age (93.4 percent and 90.6 percent, respectively), although this was more common in children in the three-to-five-year-old age range and could possibly be explained by parents seeking an "official" diagnosis of autism so that those children could be enrolled in early-intervention programs.

The methods used in the study were straightforward. Experts trained in the diagnosis of autism using the *Diagnostics and Statistical Manual IV* (*DSM IV*) went through school, hospital, and clinical records to identify children with autism. Of those 987 children, researchers were able to obtain immunization records for 660. For every autistic child researchers studied, three control children who were not autistic and were born in the same year, of the same gender, and went to the same school were also studied.

Responding to Wakefield's claim of a "regressive" form of autism, researchers attempted to identify both those children who might have developed normally for a time but then regressed and those who might have plateaued at a particular stage of development.

The results were clear. For all cases, the odds ratio was not significantly different from 1. Only in the case of children between the ages of three and five who had been vaccinated before thirty-six months was the odds ratio significant, if weak.

Using the subgroups they had defined for preexisting conditions, with regression or plateau, with or without mental retardation, the birth-certificate subgroup showed no significant odds ratios. When maternal and birth characteristics were taken into account, such as maternal age and education as well as race, no significant effect was found. In the majority of the cases of children vaccinated after thirty-six months, developmental delays had been noticed before vaccination.

Vaxxed suggests that the authors of the study were being dishonest in several ways. Brian Hooker, a heavily featured interviewee in the film, published a reanalysis in 2014 of the CDC data from the 2004 MMR study in the journal *Translational Neurodegeneration*.[3] This article was later retracted by the journal's editors when it became clear that Hooker had undeclared competing interests and that the paper had serious methodological and statistical problems.[4] Hooker's paper claimed that the original data from the 2004 study included an unreported, statistically significant increased risk for African American boys for vaccination before thirty-six months of age. This effect was based on a low number of samples and disappears when confounding factors associated with the risk of autism, such as birth weight, gathered from available birth certificates are appropriately considered.[5]

If anything, Hooker's paper demonstrates the scientific weakness of Wakefield's hypothesis, due to the degree of statistical manipulation needed to massage a small effect from the data. Hooker sliced the data into African American children and all other children, and based his conclusion on chi-squared analysis, which can't control for confounding variables, such as birth weight,[6] unlike the original paper, which did control for confounding variables.

Secret recordings of telephone calls made with William Thompson, one of the 2004 study's authors, are played in *Vaxxed* to suggest that Thompson was a whistleblower to a "cover-up" of CDC scientists who did not want the statistical analysis in Hooker's paper to be made public.

Through a lawyer, Thompson issued a statement in 2014, partially quoted here:

> I regret that my coauthors and I omitted statistically significant information in our 2004 article published in the journal *Pediatrics*. The omitted data suggested that African American males who received the MMR vaccine before age 36 months were at increased risk for autism. Decisions were made regarding which findings to report after the data were collected, and I believe that the final study protocol was not followed. I want to be absolutely clear that I believe vaccines have saved and continue to save countless lives. I would never suggest that any parent avoid vaccinating children of any race. Vaccines prevent serious diseases, and the risks associated with their administration are vastly outweighed by their individual and societal benefits.

Several of the transcripts of calls made between Hooker and Thompson were made available through Kevin Barry's book *Vaccine Whistleblower: Exposing Autism Research Fraud at the CDC*.[7] It is unclear what Thompson's precise motivation in contacting Hooker was, although it appears that they became friendly.[8] It becomes clear in the transcripts, however, that Thomson had a tendency to misinterpret scientific studies—even ones on which he was an author. Thompson's transcripts show him cherry-picking measures that appeared to be associated in studies that did not control for multiple comparisons and claiming that studies showed that they showed an association between some intervention or trait and autism. Thomson selected only those associations popping up that appeared negative, not those that appeared positive.

Part of the charge against the CDC was that a meeting was held to destroy paper documents related to the study. Although this sounds sinister, it isn't. Scientific studies often generate large volumes of data, and many institutions have time periods for which hard copies must be retained, mandated by governmental and institutional rules. After the required storage time, destroying the original data is fairly common, especially if a digital backup copy exists, as it did in the case of this study.[9] Because the digital backup of the data was not destroyed, Hooker was able to obtain the data from Thompson for his retracted reanalysis.

Finally, a charge was made that the study deviated from the analysis plan that had been set out before the study. If this occurred, it would be a cause for statistical concern because prior registration of analysis helps prevent certain kinds of statistical errors, for example, not finding the result the researcher wants and then going back to gather more data until a result is "significant." However an honest reading of the analysis plan shows that it was followed.[10] The plan stated, "The only variable to be assessed as a potential confounder using the entire sample is child's race." Hooker and Wakefield take this to mean that race was going to be tested statistically as a way to slice the data and would then be reported in the study. However, it's clear that isn't the case; race was only to be used as a possible confounding co-variable in a logistic regression—as it was used in the study.

The film centers on expanding the scientific disagreement between Thompson and the other CDC scientists writing the 2004 paper into a vast conspiratorial cover-up of data revealing that MMR causes autism, some disturbing footage of autistic children (selected for the most severe, shocking, and exploitative imagery), and a series of interviews with anti-vaccine activists. There are interviews with anti-vaccine activist Mark Blaxill; Polly and Jon Tommey, who edit the anti-vaccine magazine *The Autism File*; Sheila Ealey, who has made speaking appearances with Wakefield; Luc Montagnier, a Nobel Prize Winner, who has since endorsed various forms of quackery;[11] Doreen Granpeesheh, who previously worked with Wakefield and endorses a bogus "detoxification" theory of autism; Stephanie Seneff, a computer scientist at MIT, who makes an absurd extrapolation to claim that by 2032, 80 percent of all boys born will be autistic; Andrew Wakefield, who is the film's director (presumably interviewing himself); Del Bigtree, who is both a producer of the film and inexplicably interviewed in it; and several of the physicians from Bigtree's previous production *The Doctors*. These "fake experts" mark another of the criteria for science denial.

Hooker states regarding his son that "two weeks after his fifteen-month vaccines, then he lost all language. He lost all eye contact. You would pick him up and he would just hang limp." However, Hooker took his case to the vaccine court (see "National Vaccine Injury Compensation Program," chapter 7), and thus actual records are available.[12] The vaccine court can make awards if claimants are able either to show that an adverse event from a prespecified table occurred within a specified time period after vaccination or to show by a "preponderance of evidence" that there was a causal link between a vaccination and a specific adverse event. The standard used by the vaccine court does not include "conclusive" evidence from the medical literature, but it can include the opinion of a medical expert. *Expert* has a specific legal meaning, which isn't precisely the same as normal usage.

Due to the large volume of cases alleging autism caused by vaccination, a special proceeding was developed to try several "test cases" to test two mechanisms put forward by a group of about 180 lawyers: that the measles portion of the MMR vaccine causes autism and that thimerosal causes autism.[13] Each of the six test cases was rejected. Subsequently the majority of pending cases elected not to continue, although several went to trial, including Hooker's. Over the course of twenty-one months, Hooker's lawyers filed ten status reports with the judge as they tried to find an expert to support their case. They finally filed a report that contained a number of debunked theories from a physician with a revoked medical license. Finally, five expert reports were filed, and the case proceeded.

Medical records taken in the first year of life indicated that Hooker's son had documented developmental delays before vaccination. So Hooker's statement in *Vaxxed* that vaccination triggered his son's loss of verbal ability wasn't true.[14] Much like the CDC-whistleblower story, with a modicum of fact checking, Hooker's story falls apart.

What about Stephanie Seneff's claim that by 2032, 80 percent of male children will have autism? It's true that the number of cases of autism diagnosed has increased over time, but most scientists agree that this is an artifact rather than an actual increase in the incidence of autism. Instead, the likelihood of physicians diagnosing a child with autism has increased. We are not living through an epidemic, where the actual number of cases of autism has increased. Rather, we have started applying the term *autism* to more cases than previously would have received no diagnosis or a different diagnosis. The CDC maintains the Autism and Developmental Disabilities Monitoring Network (ADDM), which monitors the prevalence of ASD, compares its prevalence across the United States, and attempts to understand how it impacts US communities.[15] The ADDM Network reported that prevalence does appear to increase over time from 1:150 children in 2002, 1:110 in 2006, 1:88 in 2008, 1:68 in 2010, and about the same in 2012.

One component of the apparent increase has to do with racial disparities in screening and diagnosis.[16] Non-Hispanic white children are far more likely to be diagnosed with ASD than are black or Hispanic children. As time went on, these children started to "catch up" with their white counterparts. Among the dozen or so sites in the ADDM Network, there is also a large degree of variability in the estimated prevalence, indicating that cultural factors are at play in the rate of diagnosis. Likewise the rates of children without intellectual disability being diagnosed has increased, while in the past those children would not have been diagnosed.

The real conclusion to take from the ADDM Network data is that there are many children who are likely currently under-diagnosed with ASD. Better screening increases diagnosis rates. Similarly, placing better screening programs in place for the flu or childhood cancers would result in increased diagnosis rates that do not factually represent an increased prevalence.

Stephanie Seneff herself is presented as an MIT biologist, and it is true that she's a staff computer scientist at MIT; however, her biology qualifications are suspect. She earned a BS in biophysics in 1968, an MS in electrical engineering in 1980, and a PhD in computer science in 1985. Starting in 2011 she began publishing papers in biology that have been widely regarded by experts in the field as bogus. Her methods involve using computer processing of the literature in a field to generate a "story."

> It's all computer science. It's all synthesis. So basically what I do is I read papers and I process them with the computer to help me understand them and interpret them and generalize and build a story. So it's really a matter of studying. Mostly what I do now is study, and then write. Trying to understand biology. (Stephanie Seneff to AlterNet.org)[17]

Her biology papers often include titles asking leading questions, such as, "Might Cholesterol-Sulfate Deficiency Contribute to the Development of Autistic Spectrum Disorder?"; are published in low-impact, open-access, journals;[18] and posit mechanisms by which a biological event "might" occur but do nothing to test if such events actually occur. I searched three of her publications for the word *methods* and turned up nothing. A running theme in these papers is suggesting explanations for how a variety of environmental factors—such as gluten, the weed killer glyphosate,[19] or vaccines—might cause any variety of ailments. As any biologist can tell you, the ultimate arbiter of a hypothesis's value is real-world testing.

Vaxxed is capped by footage of news anchors, pundits, and entertainers discussing the 2014 Disneyland measles outbreak, as if to suggest that the potential return of measles in undervaccinated populations was an unimportant consideration to be scoffed at. This seems to be a very strange backdrop to a film that firmly takes the opinion that the currently available measles vaccine isn't safe.

By cherry-picking a single study, relying on conspiracy theories to explain the scientific consensus, relying on faulty logic, denying real experts, putting forward fake experts, and creating impossible expectations for what results research should deliver in terms of certainty, *Vaxxed* matches all of the criteria for science denial.

I watched *Vaxxed* with a friend who identifies herself as being anti-vaccine. She traced her mistrust of vaccines to a generalized mistrust of physicians. She lost faith in physicians after it took a long time for them to find the correct dose of thyroid hormone for her to take and her thyroid was removed.[20]

When *Vaxxed* ended I asked my friend if she had been convinced by the film. She said that she had. I asked what would change her mind. She said that only scientists and physicians coming out with a definitive cause for autism would convince her. This is likely to be an impossible goalpost, given the multifactorial nature of autism. Regardless of our disagreements about the film, we remained friends.

11   Too Many, Too Soon

In the two decades following Wakefield's paper, a number of other credible-seeming people have become well known for promoting anti-vaccine views. Some of them have been notable enough to warrant discussion.

In 2007 pediatrician Dr. Robert Sears, "Dr. Bob," published *The Vaccine Book: Making the Right Decision for Your Child*. In it he falls short of recommending against vaccination altogether. The book offers two schedules: one that delays receiving some vaccines, "Dr Bob's Alternative Vaccine Schedule," and another that recommends receiving only vaccines that Sears considers to be important.[1]

The book makes a number of spurious and false claims and reaches its conclusions through faulty logic. The primary problem with the reasoning of *The Vaccine Book* is the approach it takes to safety. The way that scientists evaluate safety is complex, but it's usually assumed in science that phenomena we look for aren't going to exist. With medicine there's a precautionary principle that medicines should be tested before use, just in case they cause an adverse reaction. However, *The Vaccine Book* starts with the opposite assumption—that danger may exist and that until it is tested to Dr. Bob's satisfaction, it should be assumed to exist, and even after it has been tested beyond all reasonable suspicion, it should still be assumed to exist.

Dr. Bob is the son of William Sears, "Dr. Will," creator of the Sears parenting library, which includes a number of books: *The Baby Book* (1993), *The Pregnancy Book* (1997), and *The Complete Book of Christian Parenting and Child Care: A Medical and Moral Guide to Raising Happy Healthy Children* (1997). Dr. Will is also a media personality who has appeared on many talk shows, including *The Oprah Winfrey Show* and *Good Morning America*. Three of Dr. Will's children have become physicians. One, Jim Sears, is a television personality on *The Doctors*, a spin-off of the *Dr. Phil* show, produced by Del Bigtree. Given the branding of *The Vaccine Book* and the Sears name, Robert Sears's contribution to the family business is easy to confuse with his father's.

Sears may object to being included in the same category as those who are actively anti-vaccine, since *The Vaccine Book* stops short of recommending against vaccination altogether. However, the book is dangerous in a subtler way. It borrows arguments from the anti-vaccine movement and, rather than pointing parents to good literature and the body of scientific work related to vaccines, lends those arguments the credibility of a friendly faced physician and promotes an "alternative" schedule with serious downsides and no upsides. It allows parents to feel as though they've made a rational, well-researched choice (not like those *anti-vaccine* people).

One vaccine ingredient Robert Sears focuses on is aluminum. Aluminum-containing molecules, usually alum, are used in vaccines as adjuvants. An adjuvant is something included in a vaccine that enhances the response of the immune system. Alum was first tested in the early 1920s to work with a diphtheria-toxin vaccine.[2]

Our understanding of precisely how alum enhances the immune response in vaccines is still evolving.[3] One hypothesis is known as depot formation. Researchers took skin where guinea pigs had been injected with either diphtheria toxin that was precipitated (made insoluble) or diphtheria toxoid (DT) that was soluble. This skin was homogenized (blended, basically) and injected into a new set of guinea pigs. In the newly injected guinea pigs, those injected with the skin from alum-precipitated DT became immune, but those injected with the skin from soluble-DT–injected guinea pigs did not. This led the researchers to hypothesize that the alum-precipitated DT was eliminated less quickly and that the sustained immune response is what caused immunity.[4] In this model, alum holds on to antigens in the tissue and slowly releases them. This hypothesis is not universally accepted. Others have hypothesized that injected alum recruits antigen-presenting cells, which can then trigger subsequent steps in the adaptive immune response,[5] or that alum helps antigen-loaded antigen-presenting cells to migrate to lymphoid tissues.

Regardless of the precise mechanism, or mechanisms, of action, we now have over 90 years of empirical data regarding the use of aluminum-containing compounds in vaccines. Empirically we know that it works and is safe. Specifically, the safety of each vaccine that contains aluminum (or any other ingredient) is heavily tested before being approved. The amount of aluminum per dose of vaccine in the United States is about 0.85 to 0.125 mg/dose.[6]

Sears's concern was that the aluminum in vaccines received by a child following the CDC-recommended vaccination schedule might accumulate and cause a greater effect than that from the individual doses. However, the safety profile of aluminum has been well established over decades of testing. Furthermore, there is already environmental exposure to some amounts of aluminum without ill effect. There is a small amount of aluminum present in breast milk,[7] and infant formulas contain significant amounts of aluminum.[8] Indeed the amount of aluminum in a liter of formula is comparable to the amount present in a dose of vaccine. Infants on soy-based formula take in almost twenty times as much aluminum in food during their first six months than is injected through vaccines, yet infants are successfully able to clear the excess aluminum from soy formula.[9] Sears's dislike of aluminum is not based on evidence.

For an example of the negative effects of delaying a vaccine, experts recommend that flu shots begin at six months. Not only do flu shots reduce the rate of infection, they reduce the severity of flu. Those who are infected and become sick are less likely to die or be hospitalized.[10] In 2017 in the United States there were over 80,000 flu deaths, including 180 babies, children, and teenagers.[11] This is an unusually high number. Even during the 2009 flu pandemic, nearly 60,000,000 infections led to fewer deaths. Although the number of cases of flu that lead to infant death each year are low, hospitalizations of children with flu are rarely recognized and are in the tens of thousands each year.[12] To take measles as another example, not only will children be vulnerable to infections with measles or hepatitis B, they will be able to pass measles to infant siblings, who are even more vulnerable to infection.

Sears's recommendation to space out vaccines goes against the best practices developed by the profession and does nothing to improve safety. Spacing out office visits means more office visits, with Sears's schedule requiring nineteen visits in the first five years of life. More office visits means lower likelihood of complete compliance, greater expense, and a higher workload for already overworked pediatricians, physician's assistants, and nurses. Bear in mind that all these costs in risk of infection and death, increased expense, wasted time, and increased disease burden are intended to prevent a comparatively miniscule dose of aluminum from accumulating, despite Sears's providing no plausible explanation for how it could or what harm he supposes it will cause. A tangible harm is being accepted to avoid an imagined risk.

Sears recommends against teenagers receiving the meningo-coccal conjugate vaccine. At the time *The Vaccine Book* was first written, concern had been raised from the Vaccine Adverse Event Reporting System due to five reports of Guillain-Barré syndrome shortly after receiving the vaccine. Guillain-Barré syndrome is a rare autoimmune disease. Autoimmune diseases occur when the immune system's function of determining between things that belong in your body and things that don't fails, so the immune system starts attacking tissues and cells that do belong. In the case of Guillain-Barré syndrome, the tissues being attacked are parts of the nervous system outside of the brain and spinal cord.[13] The exact causes of Guillain-Barré syndrome aren't known, so it's hard to know which proposed causes are and are not true. It is known that certain viral infections can increase risk, and the 1976 flu vaccine has been suggested to have triggered an increased risk of Guillain-Barré syndrome.[14] However, in 2012 two large and rather comprehensive cohort studies were conducted to determine if there was a link between the meningococcal conjugate vaccine and the development of Guillain-Barré syndrome. No such link was found to exist.[15] This means that parents opting out of this vaccine are accepting a risk of disease for a null benefit.

Another claim made in *The Vaccine Book* is that children vac-cinated with the Hib vaccine are at increased risk for the develop-ment of haemophilus influenzae B infection for a short period after inoculation. This suspected link was first proposed in the late

1980s after efficacy trials of early Hib vaccines were conducted. It was expected that after a single dose of vaccine, some percentage of those vaccinated would still develop a Hib infection. Studies were conducted at a number of sites, and the ability of the vaccine to protect against infection was highly variable. In Northern California, efficacy was estimated to be 68 percent based on 120,000 children;[16] 45 percent in a case-control study of children in day care;[17] 58 percent in a Minnesota-based case-control study;[18] 88 percent in Dallas County, Connecticut; and 81 percent in greater Pittsburgh.[19] In addition, several of these studies suggested a possibility that risk may increase in the week following immunization.

Two hypotheses were put forward that might have explained the cluster of cases that occurred in the first week. The first hypothesis was that the vaccine was interacting with antibodies already present in the blood and thus decreasing the number of available antibodies. A second hypothesis was that vaccination shortened the incubation time of already-infected children so that they presented symptoms sooner, although they would have become sick regardless.

In support of his concern, Sears cited three papers. The first paper, published in 1986, did not reach the conclusion that he presents it as reaching. The study selected fifty-five cases of children who had received the Hib vaccine but still caught Hib and compared the levels of antibodies in their blood to those of children who had not been vaccinated and had developed Hib infection. In 33 of these children (compared to 331 control patients) levels of the antibody against Hib were low.[20] The authors concluded that some genetic factors may be at play that caused the vaccine to fail in this case. This does not mean that the vaccine caused these children to be more prone to infection. The children in this study were *already selected* for the rare instance of the

Hib vaccine's failing to protect them from infection. This means that a far more likely explanation is that these children had low antibody levels because of some secondary (possibly genetic) factor, which is why the vaccine failed in their case. The control children were never vaccinated, so while a subpopulation may exist with the same underlying factor, that factor has not been selected for by the failure of the vaccine.

A second study examined the antibody levels in serum from children and adults for three days after inoculation with the Hib vaccine and seemed to show a 15 to 25 percent decrease in serum-antibody levels.[21] However, seven days after immunization, detectable antibody levels rose again to above the pre-inoculation value. Another study from the same year suggested that antibody levels may be depressed only in those children who already had detectable levels of antibody before vaccination.[22] Although a variety of studies suggested a possibility that there was a minor decrease in immunity for roughly seven days in children eighteen months or older who received the vaccine, the estimate of incidence with the vaccine was at most 1.6 cases/100,000, or likely lower, given the decreased prevalence of Hib in the post-vaccine era.[23] Regardless, these studies looked only at the unconjugated Hib vaccine, which was marketed from 1985 to1988, and was withdrawn because it did not produce adequate immunity in children under eighteen months of age. The current forms of the Hib vaccine, which are conjugated to adjuvants, have never been associated with an increased risk of infection. Drawing the link between a vaccine that at the time of publication had not been marketed for nineteen years and the current Hib vaccines seems a strange way to discuss risk and serves only to create needless fear.

The Vaccine Book also repeats claims about mercury in thimerosal, as well as claims that MMR vaccine may be linked to autism. I address claims of this nature at length in other chapters. Other vaccine ingredients that bother Sears include fetal bovine serum (FBS). FBS is a product used in tissue culture that is derived from cow blood. FBS contains proteins and peptides that enhance the growth of cultured cells, causing them to thrive and divide more readily in the foreign environment of a plastic dish. Although scientists have considered several alternatives to FBS,[24] they are reluctant to switch to these alternatives in many established protocols because they can change the behavior of cells. A cell line that behaves in a known and predictable way in one growth medium may behave in an unpredictable way in another medium. Sears, of course, does not attack the many other medicines that are produced similarly using mammalian-tissue culture and presumably using FBS.[25]

The primary reason cited for the concern was the possibility of mad cow disease[26] being transmitted. Mad cow disease is thought to affect the nervous system of cows, causing unusual behavior, tremors, and eventually death. No one knows for sure what causes the disease at the molecular level, although it is associated with eating feed contaminated with tissue from affected animals. One well-supported hypothesis is that the disease is caused by something called a prion.

Proteins are chains of smaller molecules called amino acids. Each amino acid in a chain has distinct properties, and when amino acids are strung together by the subcellular structures known as ribosomes, they begin to fold. The three-dimensional structure of the final protein depends on the sequence of amino acids as well as the presence of other proteins, which help them take on the correct shape. So although the one-dimensional structure of a protein, also called its sequence, might be the same, there are multiple possible three-dimensional shapes it can take on. Prions are proteins that have taken on the wrong shape and cause other proteins of the same type to take on the same wrong shape. Eventually these misfolded proteins build up and cause cells to stop functioning as they should. The accumulation of misfolded proteins in the brain leads to disruptions in its functioning and is hypothesized in mad cow disease.

Mad cow disease can be transmitted to humans, although at that point we stop calling it mad cow disease and call it variant Creutzfeldt-Jakob disease (vCJD), from which a few more than two hundred people have suffered and for which there is no known cure. Ultimately, the disease results in death. Because vCJD can be transmitted by blood product,[27] Sears's concern is that the FBS used to maintain the cells that produce the live or killed virus for vaccines may be contaminated by vCJD-causing prions. Indeed, the possibly related Creutzfeldt-Jakob disease has been known to be transmitted by contaminated doses of human growth hormone derived from human cadavers in the past,[28] although human growth hormone is no longer produced this way.

If there were an epidemic of mad cow disease in the United States, this might be a valid concern; however, there is no such epidemic. The United States has never suffered the kind of outbreak that Europe did, and Americans consume about 120 kg of meat each year,[29] second only to the United Kingdom at about 136 kilograms per person per year. Often some of this meat comes from multiple cows, yet only four cases of vCJD have been reported in the United States, all people who had lived outside of the United States.[30] If there were a widespread problem with vCJD's being spread, it would have developed through contaminated meat. (Cooking meat does not seem to prevent the spread of the disease.)

In the United States, there are recommended schedules for immunization between birth and the age of eighteen. Many workplaces and educational institutions have immunization requirements as conditions of employment and enrollment to protect their employees and students. The first recommended vaccine is for HepB at birth, followed by an additional dose after one to two months. Then, at two months, vaccines for DTaP, Hib, pneumococcal conjugate, and polio, with second doses at four months, should be given. At six months, annual vaccinations against influenza should begin (infants and the elderly are at highest risk). And, at a year, the MMR, chickenpox, and HepA vaccines should be initiated.[31]

These recommendations are considered by the Advisory Committee on Immunization Practices, which considers several factors. These factors include safety at a given age, the severity of the disease prevented by the vaccine, the infection rate in an unvaccinated population, and potential complications that might arise from application of the vaccine. The recommendations are then set by the CDC, with approval by the American Academy of Pediatrics, American Academy of Family Physicians, and the American College of Obstetricians and Gynecologists.[32] Sears goes against these recommendations on the basis of conjecture and misinterpretation of the literature.

The Vaccine Book takes great pains to appear reasonable, while muddying the water with scientific-sounding concerns that can be difficult to tease out for those without the time to seek primary sources and examine methods and conclusions carefully. Still, even some vaccine advocates will compromise by blithely saying, "It's okay to delay!," although there's no reason to delay and doing so carries serious risks.

12 Deadly Immunity

In 2005 the attorney Robert F. Kennedy Jr. wrote an article for *Rolling Stone* and *Salon*, "Deadly Immunity," which was later retracted by *Salon*,[1] but only after five corrections and six years. The piece focused on a meeting held in 2000 by the CDC at a Georgia conference center to discuss the suggestion of a risk associated with using thimerosal in vaccines. Kennedy mischaracterized it as a secret meeting, where scientists met to wring their hands over data proving the danger of thimerosal, and mined decontextualized quotes from transcripts to paint scientists and public health officials as trying to pull the wool over the eyes of the public in order to protect the interests of the pharmaceutical industry. Scientists, in his view, were conducting studies on thimerosal only to show that it doesn't work.[2] He touted studies by the anti-vaccine physician Mark Geier, who marketed a dangerous bogus autism treatment that subjected children with autism to a drug that modifies hormone levels. He also marketed possibly dangerous, and definitely unnecessary, chelation, and was stripped of his medical license in 2011 (see chapter 13).

Although *Rolling Stone* fact-checked the article, it was riddled with decontextualized quotes and factual errors. For example, quotes were taken from a scientist at the conference to imply that research into a possible thimerosal-autism link should not have been investigated and that the results should be hidden before they could be used by someone outside the group. Examining the actual transcript better reveals the context. The scientist was concerned that the results of the study and the outcome of the meeting would be misused by lawyers to profit off lawsuits that could be filed based on the study's spurious results.[3]

"Deadly Immunity" claimed that the meeting was a secret—transcripts were embargoed by the CDC; however, they were scheduled to be made public later that month. The article also claimed that much of the meeting was spent asserting a link between thimerosal and autism, and subsequently discussing how to cover up data—but that is not true. The transcript shows that the majority of participants thought that the evidence was very weak, and no discussion of how to cover it up occurred.[4] Indeed, it was clear that Kennedy mined the transcript of the meeting for quotes to make it sound like the opposite of what had actually occurred had occurred. Indeed the article even claimed that the Institute of Medicine had been paid by the CDC to cover up a thimerosal-autism link but did not present true evidence to support that claim.[5]

Salon's withdrawal of the article led to Kennedy's having difficulty in establishing credibility. He responded to the retraction on the World Mercury Project's website: "My critics have widely cited the *Salon* retraction to discredit me and my insistence that thimerosal is a potent neurotoxin that should not be in medicines [*sic*]. In recent years, newspaper editors and television producers have repeatedly cited *Salon*'s action as justification for their decisions to not run my editorials, articles and letters to the editor or to allow me to talk about vaccine safety on the air."[6] Kennedy claimed that the retraction was *Salon*'s adopting the opinion of the "pharmaceutical cartel" (see chap. 17, "Big Pharma") and that it was timed to coincide with the release of the book *The Panic Virus* by Seth Mnookin.

In 2014 Kennedy published the ironically titled book *Thimerosal: Let the Science Speak*, which took great pains to twist science in favor of the hypothesis that thimerosal in vaccines was dangerous. This is an odd argument to make given that thimerosal is only present in one current US vaccine, a flu vaccine manufactured by Noventis, which is not given to children aged four and under—well after parents and clinicians have usually noticed signs of autism. Although thimerosal is still in use in several vaccines outside of the United States, there simply isn't evidence to suggest a link between thimerosal and autism or any other neurological disorder.

Thimerosal makes use of a property of heavy metals causing them to react with certain amino acids of bacterial proteins in a way that kills bacteria. The same principle allows certain metal tools, spoons, instruments, and brass doorknobs to self-sanitize by killing bacteria. These antibacterial effects are advantageous because they allow a single vial of vaccine to be used for multiple inoculations. The controversy concerning thimerosal targeted one of the atoms present in the compound, mercury.[7] Inorganic mercury, mercury which is not bonded to carbon atoms, is known to accumulate in the brain and can cause various undesirable effects, such as nerve pain, tremors, and decreased intelligence. Some believe that the phrase "mad as a hatter" derives from mercury poisoning suffered by hat-makers who needed mercury salts to make hats, although this is likely apocryphal.

Most human exposure to mercury comes from the consumption of fish, followed by dental amalgam,[8] and occupational exposures. Other environmental sources of mercury have been slowly eliminated or phased out, such as the use of mercury in blood-pressure cuffs[9] and thermometers. Many homes, however, still have mercury switches in thermostats and pressure-control devices for gas supply. Not all sources are equal in their ability to accumulate or cause disease. Indeed, mercury can be found in multiple inorganic forms, such as vapor and mercurous and mercuric salts, and organic forms can be found in methyl, ethyl, or other configurations.[10] Each of these interacts with the body in different ways. Methyl mercury, the form mostly found in fish, for example, can be absorbed through the gut and converted into the inorganic form once in the brain. Inorganic mercury can be outgassed by dental amalgams and inhaled. When evaluating the safety of something such as the mercury in thimerosal, we need to be careful to consider the form it is in (ethylmercury), as well as dose pharmacokinetics. Pharmacokinetics is the branch of science that studies how substances move in the body once administered, what tissues they are distributed to, how rapidly they are cleared from the body, and how they are metabolized. For example, ethylmercury clears from the body about three times as rapidly as methylmercury. Pharmakokinetics gives a means to understand measures such as dose (the amount of thimerosal), the time a substance takes to break down, the rate at which it is eliminated from the body, and the rate at which it can enter other compartments, such as by passing the blood-brain barrier.

In 1999 an FDA investigation, which compared rates of cumulative ethylmercury exposure from vaccination in children in the first two years of life to guidelines for methylmercury exposure, found that the exposure to ethylmercury exceeded Environmental Protection Agency (EPA) guidelines for methylmercury.[11] Rare hypersensitivity reactions occurred with thimerosal and at extreme doses (about 1,000 times greater than early childhood exposure) were associated with neurological and renal problems.[12] Although it was unclear that thimerosal posed an actual risk, an abundance of caution won out, and vaccine manufacturers were encouraged to phase out multidose vials in favor of single-dose vials not containing thimerosal. Controversy followed this decision. On the one hand, anti-vaccine activists viewed it as vindication that thimerosal was indeed dangerous. On the other hand, those who made the decision were criticized for acting too quickly and without actual evidence of risk.

In 2003 Clarkson et al. published a review article,[13] which argued that thimerosal is quickly cleared from infants' blood in the stool and does not accumulate to unsafe levels.[14] Half-life is a pharmacokinetic property of substances that indicates the period of time after which the concentration of the substance in the body is reduced to one half the concentration it was introduced at. For example, if the half-life of substance X is one day and someone is injected with 100 mg of substance X, we will find at one day 50 mg remaining in the blood, at two days 25 mg remaining, at three days 12.5 mg remaining, and so on, until the amount remaining is undetectable. The half-life of ethylmercury in human infants is five times shorter than that of methylmercury, so it can be calculated that given a two-month period between vaccinations, mercury would not accumulate to unsafe levels.[15]

Regardless, despite no evidence of harm, the FDA recommended removal of thimerosal and started working with vaccine manufacturers to reduce levels or find alternatives.[16] As work continued to safely reduce levels, research continued to study the question of harm. In 2001 a literature review showed no evidence of harm outside of rare acute hypersensitivity.[17] In the same year, thimerosal was eliminated from newly manufactured childhood vaccines, and by 2003 the remaining vaccines had expired and were no longer usable. In 2004 a flu vaccine using thimerosal in multidose vials was recommended for children six months through twenty-three months of age, although single-dose vials are available and common.

Research continued into the safety of the additive. In 2003 two major studies were released. One, which used data from over one hundred thousand infants, showed no consistent statistical link between thimerosal exposure, and neurodevelopmental disorders.[18] Another looked at the rates of autism diagnosis in Sweden and Denmark, where thimerosal was eliminated from vaccines in the early 1990s, and found no link. At the time, many in the anti-vaccine movement were attributing a rise in autism diagnoses to the presence of thimerosal in vaccines; however, the rise in autism diagnosis occurred regardless of thimerosal's presence.[19] In 2004 the Institute of Medicine (now the National Academy of Medicine) reviewed over two hundred scientific studies that looked for a link between vaccines and autism.[20] The review concluded that there was not sufficient evidence to support either a causal link between vaccination, or thimerosal-containing vaccines, and autism. Other studies continued to examine the question, despite the lack of rigorous scientific evidence of a risk,[21] and continued to show no consistent link between early exposure to thimerosal in vaccines and developmental disorders.

Despite the astounding amount of evidence suggesting the absence of such a link, anti-vaccine activists, such as Kennedy, have continued to criticize vaccines as containing thimerosal or "toxins."

In January 2017 Kennedy announced that the then president-elect of the United States, Donald Trump, had asked him to chair a new commission on vaccines.[22] The president-elect, a former real estate developer and gameshow host, had a history of tweeting regarding the discredited vaccine-autism link, and had recently met with anti-vaccine activists.[23] The vaccine commission Kennedy had discussed with Trump has not come into existence. In effect, the federal government already has a group dedicated to ensuring the safety of vaccines, and it's not clear what a second commission would have accomplished. Trump's position was later partially reversed during the 2019 US measles outbreak.[24]

In February 2017 Kennedy, standing beside actor Robert De Niro, held a press conference and launched a "challenge," where he offered $100,000 to anyone who could "provide a study showing that it is safe to inject mercury into babies." While the challenge was effective in generating media coverage, it was unlikely to produce any serious submissions. The challenge was issued by people with "skin in the game," with an ideological commitment against thimerosal. Kennedy's past has demonstrated his willingness to play loose with the rules of scientific evidence. There is every indication that the challenge was not made in good faith. Moreover, a single study could not *prove* anything. Outside of mathematics, science does not prove or disprove, it only lends evidence for or against propositions. Proving a negative, that something does not cause *any kind* of harm, is especially difficult.

An infinite number of possible harms could be imaged from thimerosal, ranging from injection-site pain to immediate transformation into a fire-breathing dragon, and showing that none of them is possible cannot be reasonably accomplished because of the infinite number of tests that would have to be run. Compare this challenge to the one previously offered by the James Randi Education Foundation (JREF). From 1964 to 2015, the JREF offered $1 million to those who could prove they had a paranormal power or ability. Those seeking the prize would work with the JREF to develop an experimental plan that the applicants would agree to in writing, with unambiguous criteria for what would constitute a win. Of course Randi was "biased" in that he did not believe that humans could have paranormal powers, but if the agreed-upon protocol was carried out, and the criteria met, the JREF was legally obligated to have paid out. Over one thousand people were tested during the span of the challenge, and none were able to demonstrate paranormal ability.

By contrast, applicants to Kennedy's challenge did not have the opportunity to negotiate the winning criteria or agree to the win conditions. Kennedy could apparently reject the challenger outright or send the challenge to an unspecified panel. There was no reason for challengers to believe that they would get a fair chance if they sent in the fifty-dollar application fee. Finally, the challenge is a reversal of the burden of proof. The burden to prove a scientific claim always rests on the person making that claim. All who have tried to show thimerosal as causing autism have failed. A more thorough examination of the challenge was made by Craig Foster in *Vaccine*.[25]

Kennedy has continued to make news with a series of articles, a book, and various stunts; it is not clear what his goal is. Since thimerosal was almost completely removed from vaccines two decades ago, there are much more significant environmental sources of heavy-metal exposure. As the Flint water crisis showed, aged infrastructure often used lead pipes, and sites of former gas stations may still be contaminated with lead. Some populations still receive significant bioaccumulated mercury from fish. Vulnerable populations would stand to benefit greatly from highly visible activists working against actual significant sources of heavy metal exposure.

13   Ineffective "Alternatives" to Vaccination

Alongside the development of the two alternative narratives about how vaccines might cause autism, Wakefield's regressive autism and Kennedy's thimerosal, many parents of autistic children have sought "alternative" remedies to disease. Of course, where there is a market, products will be sold. The desire of anti-vaccine parents for nonvaccine remedies has fed a large market for cures and nostrums, almost none of which work, and some of which are quite dangerous in their own right. These remedies appeal not only to the antiauthoritarian desire not to let the "medical establishment" decide how people should be treated but also to beliefs that the more "natural" a treatment is, the better it is and that the longer a treatment has been in use, the better it must be. Some things found in nature are safe, others are not. Some treatments that are old are effective and safe, others are not. These are poor ways to evaluate a treatment and have led many to take up "alternative" medicine.

One such alternative proposed by anti-vaccination advocates are pox parties. Pox parties are conceptually similar to variolation in that they can introduce real immunity but different in that they result in the development of a full-blown case of the disease. During pox parties, parents deliberately expose their children to disease, hoping both to infect them with such childhood diseases as chicken pox and measles and to avoid vaccination.

Before the development of the chickenpox vaccine, when chickenpox was so widespread that nearly all children would eventually catch it anyway, the idea of getting it over with at a convenient time may have made some sense. The risk evaluation that leads a parent in the present day to take a child to such a party is premised on two erroneous beliefs: first, that vaccination carries high risk,[1] and second, that the diseases children are exposed to have a very low risk or essentially no risk at all. Both chicken pox and measles carry a risk of complications that result in further illness or death.

The deaths that occurred due to chicken pox were not and are not insignificant. About one hundred children died per year in the United States from chickenpox. This means that every year, one hundred children live, who would have died without the chickenpox vaccine. Some parents have illegally sent chickenpox-contaminated candy through the mail to allow other parents to sicken their own children.[2] This practice potentially exposes postal workers and immunocompromised children from other families to disease.

Breastfeeding (as compared to formula feeding) has occasionally been proposed to "boost" the immune systems of infants, rendering them immune to diseases. However, before the invention of formula in the late nineteenth century, the primary means of feeding infants were maternal feeding, or wet-nursing, and less commonly using animal milk.[3] If breastfeeding was sufficient to prevent every disease, there would have been no need to develop vaccination, as diseases would have been far less widespread than they in fact were. That being said, breastfeeding does provide some immune protection. The mucus membranes of a newborn are deficient in IgA, the antibody type secreted by adult humans into their guts to help protect passively against infection by foreign organisms. Other antibody types, such as IgG, are present, but in low quantities. Breast milk contains IgA antibodies that can supplement the mucus membranes of the developing gut. Although in some species there is a transfer of IgG across the gut membrane, this transfer does not occur in humans.[4] So while breastfeeding confers immune benefits in protecting infants against gastrointestinal infections, it is not a substitute for vaccination as it does not provide the kind of immune protection necessary to prevent most viral or bacterial infections.

Nosodes are a proposed homeopathic remedy that supposedly provides a degree of protection similar to that of vaccination but without any of the contents that anti-vaccine activists find objectionable, such as aluminum adjuvants, thimerosal, or actual medicine. Homeopathy was initially developed by Samuel Hahnemann at the end of the eighteenth century. It involves two ideas: a belief in the "principle of similars"—that a substance that causes symptoms similar to some ailment can cure that ailment—and a belief that this effect is amplified by serial dilution of the substance, often to the point that no molecule of the original substance exists in the preparation.[5] After many studies and systematic reviews, scientists have found no evidence that homeopathic treatments work. In addition, the proposed mechanisms of how it might work are totally implausible. Those reporting positive effects from homeopathy are mostly likely experiencing a placebo effect. Those studies that have looked at nosodes as treatments for illnesses either have been of poor quality or shown no effect or shown so small an effect as to be actually clinically unimportant. A 2015 Cochrane review of

example is ascorbic acid. Humans cannot synthesize ascorbic acid (vitamin C) so must acquire it through their diet. A modern Western diet contains more than adequate ascorbate. Ascorbate acts as an electron donor and cofactor for a number of enzymes. In cases of malnutrition wherein inadequate ascorbate is acquired through the diet, scurvy can develop with symptoms such as gum disease, weakness, bleeding, and eventual death.

At various times, claims have been made about the health effects of taking vitamin C in excess of what is necessary to prevent scurvy. Linus Pauling was a scientist whose contributions, encompassing chemistry and molecular biology, to our modern understanding of the world are hard to overestimate. In later life Pauling became an advocate for megavitamin therapy as a preventative measure or a treatment for a variety of ailments, including the common cold and cancer.[8] In 1968 Pauling presented a paper in which he coined the term *orthomolecular psychiatry* and hypothesized that various psychiatric disorders might be caused by individuals with genetic predispositions to localized vitamin deficiencies in the brain.[9] However, these ideas were tested many times and were never established to be helpful enough to become a part of medicine.[10] For the most part, excessive vitamins are simply excreted as urine; however, there are some negative side effects associated with doses of vitamins A, D, and B_6 in doses well in excess of a normal diet. Nevertheless various companies still market vitamins for various purposes they have not been shown to be effective for, such as preventing or treating the common cold.

Essential oils, or oils containing volatile compounds from plants that have strong odors, have been marketed as a means of preventing or treating disease or as a way to "detoxify" after vaccination.[11] Essential oils are a part of the quack medical practice of aromatherapy, which cannot cure or treat any disease. Some volatile plant compounds have been shown to be effective and safe for treating disease; however, when those conditions are met, they are referred to as medicine.

A variety of other quack regimens and treatments have been marketed as alternatives to vaccination, including various diets, chiropractic, and fermented cod-liver oil. None has met the standards of evidence necessary to be considered valid medical treatments. These treatments may cause no harm; however, they are often used as replacements for real medical treatment.

Where does the appeal of these bogus treatments come from? A 1998 study tested three hypotheses: that people using alternative medicine are "dissatisfied with conventional treatment, that alternative treatments offer greater personal control over health decisions, and that alternatives were more compatible with an individual's personal values, worldview, or beliefs."[12] Users of alternative health care were no more likely to report dissatisfaction or distrust with real medicine than nonusers, but were more likely to report poorer health status. However, those who used alternative medicine in place of real medicine or in addition to it were "more likely to be dissatisfied with and distrustful of standard care as well as desirous of maintaining exclusive control over their health care decisions." The study characterized users of alternative medicine generally as tending "to be better educated and to hold a philosophical orientation toward health that can be described as holistic (ie they believe in the importance of body, mind and spirit in health). They are more likely to have had some kind of transformation experience that has changed their worldview in some significant way, and they tend to be classified in a value subculture as cultural creatives." A 2008 study of Victorians in the *Australian and New Zealand Journal of*

Public Health found similarly that "the main reason people favour alternative medicine is their health-related values and beliefs."[13] Interviews with alternative medicine consumers suggested that experiences with real medicine were not a significant factor in the decision to use alternative medicine.[14] A study of the beliefs of alternative users suggests that "people use complementary medicine because they are attracted to it rather than because they are disillusioned with orthodox medicine"[15] Interview transcripts with focus groups of parents suggested that they had a strong belief in parental instinct as a decision-making mechanism and that alternative medicine offered more options.[16]

The picture this research paints is that patients seek alternative medicine not to avoid real medicine but to expand their portfolio of options and to have greater control of their own medical care. Another element that makes alternatives to real medicine superficially appealing is the placebo effect. The term *placebo effect* was introduced into the medical lexicon by English physician, Alexander Sutherland, who used it to describe hydropaths like Gibbs.[17] The placebo effect describes a remarkable fact—that patients' complaints can often be resolved without the need for actual medicine. This is seen in a number of ways. Patients given brand name pain relievers respond better than patients given identical pain relievers in plain packaging.[18] Patients treated with sham treatments often feel better, and patients who see homeopaths or chiropractors often report subjective improvements. This doesn't mean that there was no improvement, only that the improvement occurred through the placebo mechanism, and not the mechanism put forth by the practitioner.

Indeed psychological factors can have physiological effects. White-coat hypertension is a well-known example, where a patient's blood pressure can sometimes appear to be abnormally high, only when measured during a visit to a doctor's office. The clinical environment induced stress that altered the physiological value of blood pressure. So a headache patient who has a craniosacral adjustment by an osteopath has not had the sutures in their skull truly moved, but may feel better because headaches tend to improve on their own over time and because of a true physiological placebo effect.

Some have argued that placebo effects ought to be included in medicine because they can be truly effective. Many of the accoutrements of medicine—such as white coats, scientific looking instruments, and the trained-professional demeanor of doctors—are designed for just this purpose—to create a sense of meaning in medical encounters.[19] However, the placebo effect in medicine also opens ethical questions, both because it can mean lying to patients and because sham treatments can have real risks. Acupuncture carries a real risk of infection or organ puncture; infants have died or been paralyzed after "spinal adjustments" by chiropractors; Miracle Mineral Solution carries the risk of poisoning; and any placebo given in lieu of a nonplacebo treatment may not be *as* effective as the nonplacebo treatment, making it less preferable.

Merely seeking additional options doesn't mesh well with what we've seen of the anti-vaccine movement so far. While someone seeking acupuncture for back pain may not deny that pain medication and back exercises are effective treatments, the anti-vaccine movement clearly does reject real treatment. The overlap between those who deny the safety of vaccines and those seeking alternative medicine warrants additional study.

In addition to seeking alternatives to vaccination, some parents of autistic children have sought alternative treatments for autism itself. It's often difficult to discuss topics related to autism without showing preferences and making judgments about ability. The word *ableism* has been coined to allow for discussion of negative behavior associated with judgments that people make about ability, as well as to indicate how such judgments are similar to sexism or racism. *Ableism* has been defined as "the term used to describe the discrimination against and the exclusion of individuals with physical and mental disabilities from full participation and opportunity within society's systems and activities."[20] Ableism is a useful lens through which to examine much of the rhetoric generated by the anti-vaccine movement as it pertains to autism.

One of the side effects of the anti-vaccine movement is the marketing of "autism cures," which are often expensive and generally either discredited or unproven or even dangerous. Mark and David Greier marketed the "Lupron protocol," which claimed to treat autism. Lupron is a drug that mimics a hormone called gonadotropin-releasing hormone, or GnRH. GnRH is part of an axis that controls the production of the sex hormones testosterone and estradiol. Over time, the application of Lupron causes decreased sensitivity to GnRH and decreased production of these sex hormones. Lupron has been used to delay puberty in young transgender people[21] in order to prevent the development of secondary sexual characteristics that can make living in another social role more difficult. It may be used to delay precocious puberty (the onset of puberty before age eight in girls and nine in boys)[22] and has been used in patients with paraphilias or pedophilia to "chemically castrate" them by reducing levels of sex hormones.[23] Paraphilia comes in various forms, and is sexual arousal related to unusual fantasies, people, or objects.

Mark and David Geier published several papers falsely claiming that thimerosal may be associated with neurodevelopmental disorders and autism.[24] The Geiers obtained access to data from the VAERS passive surveillance system and published a study claiming increased relative risks for neurodevelopmental disorders and heart disease.[25] Their conclusions and methodology were heavily criticized by the American Academy of Pediatrics. Among the criticisms were unstated statistical methods, unverifiable results (the data they used in analysis was not made available), unrealistic assumptions about thimerosal exposure, misstatements regarding the amount of thimerosal used in routine childhood vaccination at the time of publication, failure to display their calculations, failure to show how they calculated thimerosal exposure, implication of adult heart disease as related to thimerosal based on reports from children as heart failure is often reported on death certificates but unrelated to cause of death, misleading statements about the Institute of Medicine's statements on permissible mercury exposure, and misstatements regarding the law as applied to the Vaccine Adverse Event Reporting System.[26] The Institute of Medicine convened a panel to examine the Geier's claims:

> In a report last year, a panel convened by the institute dismissed the Geiers' work as having such serious flaws that their studies were "uninterpretable." Some of the Geiers' mathematical formulas, the committee found, "provided no information," and the Geiers used basic scientific terms like "attributable risk" incorrectly.
>
> In contrast, the committee found five studies that examined hundreds of thousands of health records of children in the United States, Britain, Denmark and Sweden to be persuasive.[27]

The Geiers promoted a hypothesis that in children with autism, testosterone was interacting with mercury and that by "chemically castrating" autistic children with Lupron they could treat autism. Based on a reference in their patent application for the Lupron protocol, and the phrase "testosterone-mercury sheets," it's clear that they were misinterpreting a 1968 paper in which testosterone was crystallized with mercury in laboratory conditions in the presence of heated benzene.[28] These are not conditions that exist inside living humans. As justification for the administration of Lupron, they referenced a 1999 case report of a twenty-four-year-old man diagnosed with both autism and schizophrenia as a child and adolescent. While living at a group home, he began to develop sexual interest in young children and to masturbate publicly. Attempts were made to educate him about the need for privacy, but his public masturbation continued, and he at one point approached a group of young children in a manner that was considered to be predatory. After several other avenues were pursued, he was given Lupron to reduce his androgen levels, and his inappropriate sexual behavior was diminished.[29] This case did not specify that the symptoms of autism had diminished in the man, only his inappropriate sexual behavior, a result consistent with other uses of Lupron.

In a sixteen-part story on Neurodiversity Blog, Kathleen Seidel wrote about the Geiers, uncovering information about their research methods. These included their company's using an internal review board consisting of Mark and David Geier, a nonscientist anti-vaccine activist, a dentist, business partners, Mark Geier's wife, and an attorney involved in autism litigation. These conflicts of interest defeated the purpose of having an internal review board.

> The seven-member IRB consists of Mark and David Geier; Dr. Geier's wife; two of Dr. Geier's business associates; and two mothers of autistic children, one of whom has publicly acknowledged that her son is a patient/subject of Dr. Geier, and the other of whom is plaintiff in three pending vaccine-injury claims. The membership of the IRB

gives rise to misgivings about the independence of ethical review of Dr. and Mr. Geiers' research. Every member has discernible conflicts of interest, and none has any discernible expertise in endocrinology— expertise crucial to the competent oversight and conduct of research involving pharmaceutical manipulation of children's hormones.[30]

In 2007 an article by the Geiers was withdrawn from the journal *Autoimmunity Reviews*. The retraction followed criticism of the study's ethics.[31] Especially egregious, information about the Institutional Review Board that approved the study was submitted to the Office of Human Research Protection, by Mark Geier, fifteen months after the research had begun. To enroll children in this Lupron study, the Geiers first diagnosed them with precocious puberty, one of the few conditions for which Lupron is approved. The diagnostic criteria used do not match the criteria recommended by pediatric endocrinologists. The Geiers marketed Lupron treatment, costing thousands of dollars to the parents of children with autism, and their experimentation on autistic children continued for several years.

Those with several neurodevelopmental disabilities are often placed in a difficult position. Sexual behavior can be pathologized, and the expectations surrounding it can be difficult to agree on. In many societies sexuality is not openly discussed, and the sexual or reproductive lives of the disabled are stigmatized. Perhaps a diagnosis of autism made parents more willing to consent to treatments that modified their children's sexual development, despite putting them at greater risk of bone and heart damage. Regardless, the Lupron protocol was not based in science, and the Geiers had played fast and loose with the facts, as well as with research and medical ethics.

In part because of the work of Kathleen Seidel, in 2011 the Maryland medical board issued an emergency suspension order of

Mark Geier's medical license, for misrepresenting his credentials by claiming to be a board-certified geneticist and a board-certified epidemiologist, operating an IRB that violated regulations, and having given substandard care.[32] The medical board reviewed nine cases, finding that in six of the nine there was a misdiagnosis of precocious puberty. In three of the reviewed cases, Geier had recommended chelation therapy—the administration of drugs to remove heavy metals from the blood. Chelation therapy is only recommended when actual heavy-metal poisoning has occurred, and it carries its own dangerous side effects and risks. The nine other states in which Geier was licensed suspended his license. The suspension was upheld on appeal, and in 2012 Geier was charged with continuing to practice medicine without a license, and his licenses were formally revoked over the following months. In 2018 a judgment was made against the Maryland Board of Physicians, as in the cease-and-desist order the board issued in 2012, it publicly stated the names of medications that Geier had prescribed for himself, his son, and his wife, a violation of medical privacy.[33] Most likely this judgment will be appealed.

One problem with discussing autism cures at all is that many do not see autism as something that needs to be cured. An example sometimes given for why people with autism do not like the idea of cures comes from Iceland. In Iceland, Down syndrome has nearly been eliminated due to prenatal screening and selective abortion.[34] While it's certainly reasonable for parents to want to have healthy children, disability-rights advocates often see such practices as denying the value of the life of a person with a disability such as Down syndrome. Many disability advocates would prefer that rather than directing effort to cure autism, effort be expended to make quality-of-life improvements for people with autism. Like the Lupron protocol, numerous the time *Medical Hypotheses* was unique in being the only Elsevier journal not subject to peer review. It was dedicated to "interesting and important theoretical papers that foster the diversity and debate upon which the scientific process thrives."[43] In other words, the journal did not send papers to other scientists to review before publishing, a procedure that is an important part of the scientific quality-control process. The journal selected some odd papers for publication, for example, the 2009 paper "The Nature of Navel Fluff," wherein the author tested the hypothesis that his abdominal hair was the cause of the collection of belly-button lint.[44] In 2010 a dispute arose between Elsevier and the journal's editor over a 2009 paper that asserted that HIV does not cause AIDS. The editor's contract was not renewed, and new editorial guidelines requiring peer review were instituted.[45] The paper proposing HBOT suggested that autism is caused by inadequate blood flow to the brain. HBOT does have some real clinical applications, such as in the treatment of decompression sickness. It involves inhaling a pressurized gas mixture enriched with oxygen for some period of time.

The author of the paper, Daniel Rossignol, continued to publish on studies in which children were treated with HBOT, but the results did not support HBOT as a "cure for autism." Rather they suggested that the technique was relatively safe, and provided anecdotes to suggest an improvement in autistic behaviors.[46] Rossignol published a review that acknowledged that controlled studies did not support the hypothesis that autism symptoms improved with HBOT, but noted that in these trials there were confounders that may make the results difficult to interpret. Figures from this review include handwriting and coloring-book samples from treated children, purporting to show post-treatment improvements.[47]

Rossignol's study that received the most attention was published in 2009, the first double-blinded controlled trial of HBOT.[48]
Neuroscientist Steven Novella, a contributor to Neurologica Blog
and host of *The Skeptics' Guide to the Universe*, gave a measured
criticism of weaknesses in the study, such as allowing parents
into the chamber with children, which might alert the children
to changes in pressure, subjective measures, the short length of
the study, still-speculative mechanism, and possible bias introduced by Rossignol operating a clinical practice that offers the
treatment.[49] Others pointed out that only paired changes were
measured (changes within the treated group and changes within
the untreated group, but not differences between the treated
and untreated groups), which is an unusual method. When
appropriate statistics are applied, it appears that both groups,
including the placebo control group, improved after participation in the study.[50] Incidentally, in 2010 Rossignol was sued. The
lawsuit alleged that he prescribed potentially dangerous chelation therapy to an autistic child over the telephone without an
examination.[51]

While HBOT likely isn't very dangerous on its own, it is
expensive. It is a real therapy with actual clinical uses, so it isn't
as implausible a treatment as drinking industrial bleach, but the
evidence is not currently adequate to support its use as a treatment for autism. The cost of such therapies can be devastating
to the families of children with autism, on top of the many other
costs of care.

For a time, injections of secretin, a digestive enzyme, became
popular among parents of children with autism, after an anecdotal report showed improvements in a child given secretin.[52]
The treatment was popularized when the child's story aired on
Good Morning America and *Dateline*.[53] The sole manufacturer of

secretin quickly sold out as parents sought physicians who would prescribe secretin injections for their children. As clinical trials were carried out, it became clear that the improvements parents had observed with secretin were a placebo effect. A Cochrane review found that secretin use did not benefit autism symptoms.[54]

Another alternative therapy that has been used for autism is exorcism, a religious ritual intended to remove evil spirits. Evil spirits are not considered to be a likely cause of autism by most mainstream researchers. In at least one case, an exorcism has led to the death of an autistic child by suffocation when the would-be exorcist held the child down for hours with a knee to the chest.[55]

The Upledger Institute, named after John Upledger, promotes craniosacral therapy for the treatment of autism.[56] Upledger was an osteopath who developed craniosacral therapy based on the unproved and unlikely belief that the sutures of the skull move in rhythms due to the movement of blood or cerebrospinal fluid. When humans are born, the skull is still malleable, and rather than a single, solid skull, the neurocranium consists of a number of bones held together by fibrous sutures. The ability of the sutures to expand allows for the rapid growth in skull and brain size that occurs in the first two years of life. Sutures are sites where bone is continuously deposited and resorbed. Over time the sutures begin to grow together and interdigitate and fuse into a solid skull. The frontal suture usually fuses between the ages of three and nine months, and the remaining sutures fuse between the ages of twenty and thirty.[57] Practitioners believe that "primary respiration" occurs between sutures and can be felt and adjusted.[58] While these sutures may have some small degree of flexibility later in life, they very likely cannot be flexed by hand. There is no reliable scientific mechanism for a rhythmic movement of cerebrospinal fluid, or plausible explanation for how it "detoxifying clay baths," various diets, raw camel's milk, and essential oils. None of them have been shown to be effective treatments for the symptoms of ASD. Parents, although undoubtedly seeking the best for their children, have been sold a variety of expensive and sometimes dangerous treatments. Often because many of the symptoms of ASD change with time, and are difficult to measure objectively, anecdotal improvements or changes are incorporated into stirring testimonials without scientific weight.

Many advocates have criticized the charity Autism Speaks on a number of grounds. The organization was established in 2005 but did not include any people with autism on its board of directors until 2015.[62] The charity's budget was largely focused on research intended to prevent autism. This prevention was most likely to be in the form of prenatal screening, which would allow parents to perform selective abortion of children likely to have symptoms of autism.[63]

In 2009 the executive vice president of Autism Speaks, Alison Singer, resigned over the organization's decision to continue funding research looking for a link between vaccinations and autism.[64] However, since 2017, Autism Speaks has reversed course, offering the following statement on their website:

> Each family has a unique experience with an autism diagnosis, and for some it corresponds with the timing of their child's vaccinations. At the same time, scientists have conducted extensive research over the last two decades to determine whether there is any link between childhood vaccinations and autism. The results of this research is clear: Vaccines do not cause autism. The American Academy of Pediatrics has compiled a comprehensive list of this research.[65]

Others have pointed to the language used by Autism Speaks as being potentially stigmatizing for people with autism, leading to the exclusion or mistreatment of people with autism. This has led to complaints that an advocacy group for people with autism is primarily composed of parents of children with autism, who may have goals conflicting with those of people with autism themselves.[66]

While some of the symptoms sometimes associated with ASD can be ameliorated with speech therapies, augmented communication, and individual education plans, cures marketed for autism are universally not science based. Such "cures" can victimize people with autism by exposing them to risky treatments, poisonous drinks, or expensive and ineffective treatments.

14 Social Media, "Fake News," and the Spread of Information

While traditional media helped spread misinformation, after Wakefield's paper was published, in the forms of books, newspaper and magazine articles, and television shows, increasingly, social media and other new forms of communication have supplanted traditional media as primary means of disseminating anti-vaccine misinformation. While eighteenth-century anti-vaccine activists distributed pamphlets and held rallies, modern anti-vaccine activists have access to cell phones, Facebook, Twitter, Snapchat, and other forms of social media. However, while the speed and ease of communication has greatly improved in the last decades, the safeguards to ensure the information being transmitted is good has not. Communication technology has changed rapidly in the last century, moving from print journalism, radio, television, to the early internet, and social media. Social media make use of direct person-to-person communication, absent centralized gatekeepers that previous means of communication had.

Those who follow US politics have become familiar with the term *fake news*,[1] an accusation that has been leveled at both reliable journalists, who honestly seek to present the truth in their writing, and those seeking to destabilize the US government through deliberate propaganda campaigns. Scientists have begun to study the phenomenon of fake news[2] and how it propagates. Fake-news stories are those that have the appearance of being real-news stories but do not have the editorial supervision of traditional news sources and do not adhere to journalistic norms for verifying information before disseminating it. This is not an unprecedented phenomenon. In 1835 the *New York Sun* boosted its circulation by publishing a series of fake-news stories describing bizarre and incredible life discovered on the moon.[3] In May 2019 a fake-news story spread online in which Nancy Pelosi, Speaker of the House of Representatives, had been slowed down to make her appear to be drunk and have slurred speech. While previous changes in dominant forms of communication have elicited fears, never before have individuals had the power to reach as many people as established news sources have had. Most US adults now get at least some of their news through social media.[4]

The reach of fake-news stories is significant. In the lead-up to the 2016 US election, fake-news articles were read an estimated 760 million times and shared 38 million times.[5] More than being widespread, fake news potentially reaches more people more easily than does real news. On the social-media platform Twitter, fake-news stories propagate "farther, faster, deeper and more broadly" than true stories.[6] False stories reached more people, jumped from more users, had greater success going viral, and were 70 percent more likely to be retweeted than were true stories. Those who primarily consume news online are more likely to believe in 9/11 conspiracy theories.[7] This is a concern because 80 percent of internet users search for health information online.[8]

The same principles that allow fake news to spread more rapidly and deeply than real news does online apply as well to anti-vaccine conspiracy theories and medical advice. These conspiracy theories decrease the likelihood of those exposed to them to want to vaccinate.[9] Such beliefs are widespread and not dependent on political affiliation.[10] A large fraction of websites presented by search engines can be anti-vaccine, and there is a high probability that someone seeking information on vaccines will encounter anti-vaccine websites;[11] as of 2008 over half of the search results returned for "vaccine safety" and "vaccine danger" were inaccurate.[12] About one-quarter of these websites aspire to claims of authority by imitating those of official organizations or by citing dubious literature, and many frame vaccination as a "debate" occurring within the medical community and offer "unbiased" information. Many make appeals to emotion, telling personal stories of those supposedly harmed by vaccines, and establish those who advocate for vaccination as adversaries, liars, shills, or victims of manipulation. Ironically, these websites often portray themselves as boldly presenting the truth amid a culture of lies, cover-ups, and appeals to the naturalistic fallacy.[13] The decline in infectious diseases is attributed to other (often unexplained) causes, and the tragedy and severity of vaccine-preventable illnesses is downplayed.

Anti-vaccine claims on the internet are not static. They respond to changing news stories and the development of new rhetorical techniques.[14] An analysis of vaccine-opposing websites showed a slight decline in the number attributing vaccines with causing a variety of illnesses from nearly 100 percent to about 76 percent. Arguments based on civil liberties declined from about 80 percent to about 40 percent of websites. Promotion of "alternative" treatments declined from 45 to 70 percent[15] to 20 percent. Claims of financial conflicts declined from 88 percent to 52 percent. The number of websites promoting conspiracy theories increased slightly. Mention of "aborted fetal tissue" also declined.[16] Two new themes were noted: falsifying the threat of disease and using testimonials by those claiming expertise. A 2009 survey of over 175,000 Canadian internet users during the swine-flu pandemic found that only 23.4 percent of users considered the H1N1 vaccine to be safe,[17] showing how rapidly anti-vaccination rhetoric can respond to current events. Remarkably, despite the tactics of anti-vaccination websites adapting over time, the overall messages being spread fall into the same basic categories used by John Gibbs in the 1850s.[18] The themes of personal liberty, fears of body pollution, and distrust of the government and scientists are still used more than a century and a half later.

YouTube, the world's largest video-sharing site, shows how anti-vaccine rhetoric has permeated the public discourse; in an analysis, nearly a third of vaccine videos analyzed carried a negative message about vaccination.[19] As of 2012 the majority of videos about the HPV vaccine were negative in tone[20] and had more "likes" than positive videos. As more people stop using cable and broadcast television as sources of entertainment, personally made videos and testimonials will become a larger and important means of receiving and processing information.

Pinterest is a website that allows users to collect images and videos on "pinboards" by topic. A 2015 study examined the way vaccines are portrayed on Pinterest. Seventy-four percent of pins studied were classified as anti-vaccine.[21] Pinterest is one of the few platforms with a policy that specifically bans information it deems harmful, including anti-vaccination advice. According to Pinterest's community guidelines in 2018, "We don't allow advice when it has immediate and detrimental effects on a pinner's health or on public safety. This includes promotion of false cures for terminal or chronic illnesses and anti-vaccination advice." However, a search on the Pinterest search engine shows that a majority of pins for the word "vaccination" are anti-vaccine.

The social network Facebook also serves as an incubator of anti-vaccine beliefs, hosting many anti-vaccine groups. Some state their purpose outright; others attempt to appear moderate by presenting a false equivalence and offering seemingly neutral information. These groups include the Vaccination Re-education Discussion Forum with 121,000 members, the Vaccine Education Network: Natural Health Anti-Vaxx Community with 32,000 members, and Vaccine Injury Stories with 22,000 members, as well as Vaccine Haters, Vaccine Research Society, Vaccines Exposed, United against Vaccines, Vaccines—The Lies, Vaccine/Immunization Common Sense, Parents against Vaccination, Vaccine Danger, Educate before You Vaccinate, Vaccine Abolition Society, Parents Questioning Vaccines, Pet Parents against Vaccination & Over Vaccination, Vaccine Truth Movement, and The Vaccine Gamble—all with thousands or tens of thousands of followers. The anti-vaccine page Stop Mandatory Vaccination has been liked 117,000 times, the Vaccination Information Network (VINE) has been liked 148,000 times, and The Truth about Vaccines has been like 138,000 times. These webpages share personal testimonials and memes intended to discourage vaccination. In March 2019, in the midst of a US measles outbreak, Facebook pledged to address anti-vaccine content on its platform, but progress has been slow[22] and, rather than banning anti-vaccine groups, will likely take the form of automated links to better sources where anti-vaccine content is shared and links to better content for users searching the platform for accurate information.

One way that anti-vaccine content has been shared is through memes. The word *meme* was coined by the biologist Richard these bans triggered concern that large social-media companies were capable of censoring free speech.

Freedom of speech is generally recognized to be freedom from government restrictions on speech, but most recognize that freedom of speech has limitations. Under this strict definition, the loss of the use of a platform such as Mailchimp is not a restriction on freedom of speech. Freedom of speech is, however, also a cultural phenomenon.[30] Without that culture, legal and institutional protections for speech are in many ways symbolic. Seeing speech punished can lead to self-censorship and fear. Large media companies control significant avenues by which we communicate, so their actions are deserving of scrutiny. The bans on InfoWars's content occurred within a larger and ongoing cultural debate over the limits of free speech. Protests on college campuses have caused controversial talks to be canceled. Protestors argued that the protests were justified by a "higher moral responsibility to prevent marginalized groups from being victimized by hate speech." This was against those who saw themselves as representing "the students' right to hear these speakers."[31]

Previous forms of mass media had even stricter corporate control. Operating a television station was inaccessible to most people, and most news broadcasters adhered to editorial guidelines and instructions from the companies that owned them. Likewise, print media were generally difficult to produce and distribute. The existence of editors allows journalistic standards to arise by limiting the kinds of content that received widespread distribution. Despite this, fringe publications still existed. Jones was using those social-media platforms to advocate for violence, which has long been recognized as a reasonable kind of speech to restrict. However, the interface between platforms that elevate individual voices and the social responsibilities of the corporations that control those platforms raises important questions that have yet to be addressed.

Misinformation about diseases and public health risks is also readily available on the internet.[32] Often the most easily available information is misleading. A survey of information about the Zika virus available through popular search engines showed that a variety of conspiracy theories and misinformation appeared among the first results (such as fear of genetically modified mosquitoes and a belief that the Zika virus was a plan to undermine national sovereignty). By looking at the spread of anti-fluoridation misinformation, researchers concluded that social relationships may be more important for spreading misinformation than is the scientific content of such information.[33] This finding is consistent with culturally competent means of addressing vaccine hesitancy as being most effective. Rather than evaluating the truth of claims, we evaluate the trustworthiness of sources based on our relationship to those sources.

Social networks fundamentally extend the human ability to gossip. Although the word *gossip* can have negative connotations, it is an important means for learning about social relationships and the day-to-day events in the lives of people around us.[34] However, while this is an effective method for gaining information about the world as it pertains to social relationships, its reliability breaks down when ascertaining information about the physical world, as in "What actually happened? What is the actual truth?" Thus, the means by which nonscientists and scientists evaluate risk and truth are nonoverlapping. It isn't that anti-vaccine activists usually dismiss the determinations of scientists outright, or are unwilling to consider scientific evidence, but rather that the kinds of scientific evidence they accept and repeat, and those experts they listen to, are selected by criteria different from those used by actual scientists.

Cultural cognition is a hypothesis that may help explain some of this disparity. This hypothesis states (in summary) that we assess risks not based on accumulated facts and knowledge but, rather, in line with our cultural preconceptions and biases. For example, in a 2012 study, it was shown that those with the highest scientific literacy and technical-reasoning ability were likely to be most polarized on the issue of climate change.[35] This finding suggests that inadequate knowledge of science is a secondary factor to this kind of scientific risk determination. A 2010 survey studied the perceived risks of the HPV vaccine with reference to two phenomena, biased assimilation and the credibility heuristic. Biased assimilation refers to the tendency of those who hold strong opinions on complex issues to examine empirical evidence in a way that is biased toward confirming their prior beliefs and to more critically evaluate evidence that challenges those beliefs.[36] The credibility heuristic refers to the tendency to assess information as being more credible when it comes from sources perceived to share group membership with the evaluator.[37] The authors hypothesized that a person's position on mandatory HPV vaccination would depend on perceived in- or out-group status of the person providing the information based on cultural cues. The identity of those making the argument was predictive of the likelihood of a person to agree with the argument.[38]

Some have suggested that cultural cognition may be only one of several factors that go into risk evaluation. Regardless, there are a number of cognitive biases that make group membership and personal relationships important determinants of how human beings perceive information. This is illustrated by the study of a

1951 football game between the Dartmouth Indians and Princeton Tigers.[39] The game was rough and injuries resulted. When
students were later surveyed, of one hundred Dartmouth students, fifty-three believed that both sides started rough play, and
only thirty-six believed that Dartmouth alone was responsible.
Of one hundred Princeton students, eleven believed that both
started rough play and eighty-six believed that Dartmouth was
responsible. Although only one game was played, and a series
of events occurred, the subjective perception of those events
depended heavily on the group to which an observer belonged.
This effect is termed *selective perception*.

As human beings we have difficulty assessing our own level of
knowledge and competence. This has been termed the Dunning-
Kruger effect. The psychologists David Dunning and Justin Kruger conducted four studies in which participants were presented
with tasks that required knowledge in humor, logical reasoning, or English grammar, and compared the participants' self-
assessment of their abilities to their actual scores. In each case,
participant's scores diverged most from their self-assessment
among those with the lowest scores. Conversely, those with the
highest scores tended to underestimate their abilities.[40] Several
explanations have been offered for this effect, including a lack
of metacognitive ability among the incompetent; the inability
to make accurate "social comparisons"; a tendency to compare
one's own ability to that of others; and the simple possibility
that the less you know, the less likely you are to know how
little you know. Dunning and Kruger's work has been widely
misrepresented as meaning that the less competent one is, the
more competent one believes oneself to be, which is not quite
accurate; their work showed a positive correlation between perceived ability and actual score. Alternative explanations for these

phenomena have included regression to the mean,[41] which is a statistical tendency of groups selected for one trait to be average on other traits, and the possibility that both high and low performers have a similar capacity to assess their abilities, but only a few high performers exist. This makes it difficult for low performers to see examples of high performance against which to judge themselves.[42]

Assessment of bias in others is another area of human perception prone to biases[43] that may in some way explain how anti-vaccine information is perceived online. We tend to see ourselves as being less affected by cognitive biases than others are. Others' motivations are unknown and thus subject to scrutiny. However, we can introspect on the nature of our own motivations, regardless of whether that introspection reaches the correct conclusions.[44] Unable to peer into others' minds, we must rely on hypotheses and theories as to their motivations.

In some ways we can build protections against these kinds of biases into how we function in our lives. For example, Robert's Rules of Order—the set of rules for parliamentary procedure that govern most proceedings in government, business, academia, and nonprofits—specifically ban calling into question the motivations of another member of a deliberative body.[45] Reasoning that "Person X is a scientist, so they're motivated by big-pharma money" is an example of how this kind of biased reasoning might act in vaccine discussions. The reverse is of course also true. Vaccine advocates engaging in online discussion may presume bad faith, where none exists, on the part of the vaccine hesitant.

In many ways science has not yet caught up to social media in its ability to disseminate information. Many scientists prefer traditional media sources.[46] Our means of communicating scientific information are still mostly modeled after means of communication that are now largely dead. Scientific journals often include short scientific reports in a format similar to that of a written letter. Printed scientific journals themselves are also artifacts of a past era. The majority of scientific journal articles are now read in digital formats, but publishers often still charge extra for color figures. At the same time that we publish within the walled garden of scientific research, scientific stories that are picked up by the popular press and social media often aren't represented in a way that is accurate to the nature of the research or how well it represents the field as a whole.[47] Scientific journal articles are also often kept behind paywalls, and so are available only to those with access to institutional subscriptions, and are often thick with discipline-specific language, stuffed with jargon that makes them difficult to understand for those who aren't members of the specific scientific field that the papers come from.

The social costs of engaging with the anti-vaccine movement are quite real. Holly Griffeth, a NASA engineer and a friend of the author, shared via social media a typical story of an emotionally charged family interaction relating to vaccination. "Recently I went out to eat with my mom, my cousin, and her husband. They had recently had their first child. Somehow the discussion turned to vaccines and they mentioned they weren't sure about them. This was somewhat mind-blowing, as I considered her reasonably intelligent. She said that she had talked to 'a few friends' who said that their kids started acting completely differently after getting the MMR vaccine and they were afraid of autism. That was her empirical evidence." Holly had never realized that there were people in her life who actively opposed vaccination. She decided to share pro-vaccination memes on Instagram. "I never tagged her in anything or called her out, I didn't even follow her on FB. She easily could have done the same but she made a big deal about it. This pissed off my mom, who accused me of 'attacking her family,' which set off a whole other round of craziness. Recently I posted something on IG about vaccines and she replied angrily, telling me to shut my mouth and that her son would NOT get the MMR—I don't think I even realized she followed me. So that resulted in me blocking her from IG and FB and my mom from FB. This was 6 months ago."

Holly's experience is typical of social-media interactions surrounding vaccines. Neither party was willing to give an inch, and neither party did. Her cousin had received information from trusted people in her real-life social network and based her vaccination decision primarily on her trust in those friends.

Because of the mismatching expectations, expertise, and understanding of science between vaccine advocates and the vaccine hesitant, social-media discussions of scientific topics often derail and leave both these types of participants emotionally charged but unmoved in opinion.

That doesn't mean that social media needs to be abandoned as a means of communication. Facebook has an available audience several orders of magnitude larger than that of traditional means of scientific communication.[48] Hundreds of millions of tweets are posted daily, and hundreds of millions of people use social-media platforms. Like it or not, these platforms have become the de facto means by which most nonscientists receive and access information about scientific discoveries. Internet communication can even lead to positive outcomes. Use of the internet increases positive attitudes about science overall,[49] and access to science blogs can help address knowledge gaps across social classes.[50]

However, there's value in addressing misinformation when it is encountered on Facebook and Twitter. Exposure to misinformation potentially harms public health efforts. Vaccine-critical web pages can quickly increase the perception of vaccine risk[51] and decrease the likelihood of parents to vaccinate.[52] The majority of parents forgoing vaccination cite the internet as a major source of information, despite these parents remaining a minority of parents overall. Although vaccination rates remain high, providing access to good information may prevent enclaves of low vaccine coverage and more outbreaks similar to the Disneyland and Minnesota measles outbreaks.

Since at least the early 2000s, attempts have been made to correct the record online by providing factual resources to counter anti-vaccine information. These work on an information-deficit model of science communication. The information-deficit model suggests that people with negative attitudes on scientific topics are simply lacking adequate information and that the provision of enough information will change the polarity of their attitude.[53] However, the correlation between science knowledge and attitudes toward science and technologies (such as vaccination) is positive but weak.[54]

An alternative model for how people process information about science is the low-information rationality model. In this model the benefits of becoming an in-depth expert in scientific and political topics are low, and human beings tend to be parsimonious with effort. To make up for this, we use heuristics, or rules of thumb, to develop "gut reasoning" about various topics.[55] In this model, information does matter—as the less information a person has available to them when making a decision, the more likely they are to rely on heuristics.[56] Two mechanisms by which media or social media might influence attitudes toward vaccination are cultivation and framing.[57]

Cultivation refers to the ways in which frequent exposure through media can cultivate particular attitudes about a topic. For instance, frequent exposure to news reports of violence might cultivate a belief that violence is more frequent than it actually is. Likewise, frequent exposure through social media to false information about vaccine safety might cultivate a negative attitude about the safety of vaccines.

Framing exploits preexisting associations to create new associations. For instance, framing a news story about vaccines with an image of a screaming child, upset at having to get a shot, brings with it negative associations of unhappy children or children in pain.

Rather than a battleground, social media can be a powerful tool for scientists and public health advocates to reach the vaccine hesitant, so long as advocates are conscious of how they are framing information, not simply trying to overwhelm anti-vaccine activists with information, and telling a positive story about why vaccination is the correct choice for them.

15   Escalation of Commitment

The pathway to go from a curious person seeking information on the internet to an active member of an anti-vaccine group, sharing or generating memes, sending physicians death threats, or spilling menstrual blood on state legislators is not a clear one.

How do people become entrenched in anti-vaccine views? There are a number of hypotheses that seek to explain how behavior can become more entrenched over time and how groups can become more polarized.

When people become committed to courses of action, they rarely rationally reevaluate their commitments to action at each step and rarely step back when confronted by a mistake. Graduate students, having invested six years in obtaining an advanced degree, will often continue seeking a faculty job, even though the odds of getting a tenure-track faculty job decrease every year. Stockholders may continue to buy shares even after their price has fallen several times. Couples may persist in romantic relationships well after the "spark" is gone. A nation may double down on its commitment to a losing war so that its soldiers cannot be said to have "died in vain." Business executives are more likely to allocate money to a failing division when they themselves made the initial investment in that division.[1]

Several hypotheses may partially explain these human behaviors. One is that when people make decisions, they simply do not like to admit that they were wrong. Another is that people tend to double down on investments they view as moral imperatives because they want to see themselves as moral.[2] Another is that we value self-consistency and will pursue behavior that allows us to see ourselves as consistent, even if that behavior is not necessarily rational.[3] Those who identify strongly with a group will also more strongly escalate commitment to a group's decision when it fails,[4] hence our commitments to belonging in groups can also influence us to overcommit resources to failing ideas.

A related idea is called the sunk-cost fallacy, or the gambler's fallacy. If we choose to wait for a bus instead of taking a half-hour walk, we are prone to continue waiting, even if the bus is so late that it gets us to our destination later than if we had given up and started walking there instead. Gamblers will continue putting money into a game they are losing in the belief that they must recoup the money they have lost with an upcoming "big win." Gamblers will sometimes become destitute, chasing sunk costs by continuing to gamble—so strong are the biases that lead us to chase wins.

Belonging to groups can also make us more committed to the decisions of those groups, and make us take up more polarized positions than those we would have been inclined to without the group's influence.[5] Social media, although it has exposed us to more viewpoints than ever before, also allows us to become *more entrenched* in our viewpoints.[6]

Several causes may underlie this group polarization. We may express stronger views to be perceived in a positive light by the group. In this social-comparison model, we are constantly seeking to achieve group harmony and status within a social group.

In another model, groups allow us to share information, in ways that are biased. When a group discussion occurs, the group is more likely to bring up arguments favoring one viewpoint. If those arguments are novel, we add them to our internal model of the issue and formulate a viewpoint that is influenced to include more arguments in one direction. Individuals with less entrenched views may be driven away from groups as their views become more extreme.

People who are initially agnostic toward vaccines, but who are exposed to members in their community who oppose them, may start to express anti-vaccine views to fit in with their community. Being surrounded by those with anti-vaccine views, they may be exposed to more anti-vaccine arguments over time and thus develop a mental model of vaccination that is based largely on arguments against vaccination that they have been exposed to through their group membership. Thus, over time their views become more solidified.

16   Religion and Vaccine Hesitancy

Laws vary with regard to vaccination, by country and by state. Most states require that children be up to date on their vaccine schedule in order to be allowed to attend schools or day care centers. However, some states provide for exemptions to this. The first category are legitimate medical exemptions. These would be granted to children who have compromised immune systems, allergies to a vaccine component, or some other medical reason for which they cannot be vaccinated. However, in many cases, these exemptions have been exploited. Parents have shared the names of pediatricians willing to sign exemption documents— for a fee. The next category are religious exemptions. Because religion often occupies a privileged status in society, many states have allowed parents to exempt their children from vaccination on religious grounds. However, this kind of exemption may also be exploited.

The religions of the world are diverse, representing many different supernatural explanations for the nature of reality, beliefs, and practices, so it is difficult to make blanket statements about whether a religious objection to vaccination can ever accurately reflect a person's religious beliefs. However, the majority of world religions don't hold an objection to vaccination as actual official belief. Because many states allow for religious exemptions to vaccination, in effect, religious belief becomes a convenient scapegoat for vaccine objections, especially in jurisdictions without personal philosophical exemptions.

The explanations for these objections are as varied as the religions in the world,[1] and even within some religions, such as Christianity, there are multiple sects with differing views. Conversely, religious leaders can play a role in helping communities to achieve high levels of vaccine coverage, as seen after the recent Minnesota measles outbreak and among Buddhist women who were early proponents of variolation.[2] However, religious leaders who are in favor of vaccination often do not preach its use.[3]

Moreover, it is very difficult to define which religious beliefs are legitimate, or illegitimate. Most would not argue that a religious belief is only legitimately held if it is endorsed by a major religious organization or denomination. However, based on the accounts of former anti-vaccine parents, it is clear that many requested religious exemptions, despite not holding a religious belief with regard to vaccination. The difficulty in distinguishing between a "true" religious belief and one that was manufactured to bypass rules is exactly the problem states face by allowing religious exemptions to vaccination. While that demarcation is too difficult to make, we can ask two related questions: Do any religions with large numbers of followers prohibit vaccination? And should states allow religious exemption?

Studies of how common religious exemption is are rare. A 2013 study examining the rates of religious exemption in New York State from 2000 to 2011 indicated that in 2011, although very few sought religious exemptions, only about 0.4 percent of parents, this number was nearly double that of the 0.23 percent of parents seeking religious exemptions in 2000, suggesting a potential rise in this class of exemption.[4] These numbers do not include homeschooled children, a growing group, and some rural counties had a greater than 1 percent exemption rate.

Deliberate exemption on religious grounds may not be the only way that religion influences vaccination decisions. Religion may bias parents against certain vaccinations, without leading them to seek an explicit exemption on those grounds. HPV vaccines, for example, are not required for school attendance and would not show up in studies based on religious exemptions. Parents with frequent attendance at religious services are less likely to vaccinate against HPV, while Catholic parents are more likely than nonaffiliated parents to have vaccinated.[5] Often religion is presented to medical providers by parents as their reason for requesting vaccine exemptions.[6] In addition, the means by which vaccines are produced has resulted in objections by some on religious grounds. Some vaccines are produced in cell lines derived from human fetal tissue, leading to objections from religious leaders who dislike the use of tissue derived from a human fetus, and other religious leaders have objected to vaccines produced with cow tissue or porcine tissue.

In the past decade, measles outbreaks have been reported in several countries with sizable Muslim populations, including Pakistan, Malaysia, Nepal, Cameroon, Nigeria, South Sudan, Guinea, and Egypt.[7] In 2009 the swine flu, H1N1, was classified as a pandemic with an unusually virulent strain, especially among the elderly. Concurrent to the height of the outbreak, the Saudi government prepared for the 2009 (1430 AH) hajj season.[8] Since the hajj involved the movement of approximately 2.5 million people, the possibility of influenza being transmitted was high. Among National Guard workers assigned to the hajj, only 46.8 percent accepted vaccination.[9] Although the Saudi

Health Ministry recommends vaccination to pilgrims,[10] the
rate of flu vaccination has been low in most years. So in 2004
vaccine hesitancy was a valid concern; pilgrims spread polio to
several countries while attending the hajj.[11] Different countries
responded to the risk differently. While Egypt and China, for
example, required that pilgrims be vaccinated before departure,
the United States did not. Despite the logistical challenges, the
2009 hajj was successful.

A significant challenge to views on vaccination in some
Muslim-majority countries came in 2011, when it came to light
that Dr. Shakil Afridi had aided US intelligence agencies in track-
ing down Osama bin Laden by leading a HepB-vaccination campaign that collected DNA.[12] When news came out about this
campaign, public health officials were horrified.[13] There was
already opposition to vaccination efforts in the region due to
conspiracy theories about vaccination being used to sterilize the
local population. Only three countries still have polio transmission, Afghanistan, Pakistan, and Nigeria, all targets for polio-
eradication efforts. Taliban commanders in Northern Waziristan
have spoken out against polio vaccination.

Following these revelations, in 2012 nine polio-vaccine workers, mostly women, were murdered, shot by men on motorcy-
cles,[14] most likely as a consequence of the fake polio-vaccination
campaign. Then in 2013 nine more polio-vaccine workers
were killed in Nigeria, mostly women, shot in the back of the
head.[15] Nigeria had a history of vaccine opposition. In 2003 an
eleven-month ban was placed on polio vaccination after a Muslim scholar feared that polio vaccination might be a US plot[16]
and that the vaccines might be contaminated with "antifertil-
ity drugs, contaminated with certain viruses that cause HIV/
AIDS, contaminated with Simian virus that are likely to cause

cancer."[17] In 2016 fourteen people were killed in an explosion near a polio center, mostly police officers protecting the center, and later that year seven vaccine workers were killed in an attack. In early 2018 a mother-daughter vaccination team was murdered in Pakistan, and in 2018 two more vaccine workers were murdered in Pakistan.[18] The mistrust engendered by the use of a polio-vaccination campaign as a front has likely slowed the efforts to eradicate polio worldwide. In 2018 there were thirty-three cases of wild polio virus and seventy-five cases of circulating vaccine-derived polio virus.

In August 2018 the Indonesian Ulema Council declared the MMR vaccine to be haram (forbidden by Islamic law), leading to concerns that religiously conservative Indonesians may eschew vaccination, as well as a rush to develop an MMR vaccine that did not contain incidental porcine products.[19] Conversely, a number of gatherings of Muslim scholars have determined that vaccination is acceptable in Islam and that porcine gelatin in some vaccines is acceptable. Meanwhile an outbreak of measles is ongoing in Indonesia as of 2018.[20]

These incidents aside, the majority of Muslim scholars support vaccination, and the majority of Muslims have no problem with immunization. Worldwide, religious leaders have been critical aids to vaccination efforts and the efforts to eliminate smallpox and polio.

There were early concerns among Jewish scholars that vaccination may not be kosher (adhering to specific Jewish dietary laws); however, a number of rabbis and scholars have written opinions stating that vaccination is allowable or even a mitzvah, or religious duty. Dietary restrictions are commonly understood to apply to oral consumption. In the past Shabbat restrictions have been placed on vaccination in some Orthodox communities;

however, this is only one day a week, and Jews were encouraged get vaccinated on other days. The Orthodox Union and the Rabbinical Council of America have strongly urged vaccination.[21]

The 2019 US measles outbreak had about half of its cases occur in Rockland County, New York, and Brooklyn, New York, in its Orthodox Jewish communities.[22] Many of these cases were in private religious schools that did not have a vaccination requirement. Following the outbreak, tens of thousands of vaccines have been administered in Rockland County and thousands more in Brooklyn, bringing vaccination rates above 95 percent, in hopes of slowing the spread of measles. A forty-page pamphlet had circulated within the Orthodox community called *The Vaccine Safety Handbook*, published anonymously and containing misinformation.[23] Anti-vaccine activists have held rallies leading up to and in the midst of the outbreak, including people such as Del Bigtree, who produced *Vaxxed* and runs an anti-vaccine YouTube channel.[24] Also present have been Orthodox protestors in favor of vaccination.

The form of Christianity known as Catholicism has stated opposition to abortion, which raised concerns among some followers about the use of vaccines produced in cell lines derived from tissue extracted from aborted fetuses. However, a statement issued by the Pontifical Academy for Life said (in summary) that Catholics should seek alternative forms of these vaccines, and in cases where such forms are not available, they are permitted to be vaccinated with them, although that is not an endorsement of the means of production.

Jehovah's Witnesses practice a form of Christianity. Their organizing body instructs followers to refuse whole blood transfusions, as well as certain blood products, based on the group's interpretation of religious texts. In recent decades these restrictions have loosened somewhat to allow certain blood products. In the 1920s through the 1940s, the Watch Tower Bible and Tract Society banned members from vaccination under penalty of excommunication. In 1952 this restriction was loosened, and over the decades a neutral stance has been taken.[25]

The Amish and Hutterites, smaller Christian subtypes, do not proscribe vaccination; however, their vaccination rates are variable but somewhat low.[26] Indeed, surveys of Amish households have shown that vaccination is not universally rejected and that the primary reason nonvaccinating Amish families do not vaccinate is not religious.[27]

Like other Christian groups, the majority of mainline Protestant Christian churches do not have religious objections to vaccination, although this is a broad category, so smaller groups may have individual differences and individual religious leaders may occasionally take an anti-vaccine stance.

The Church of Christ, Scientist is a form of Christianity founded in the late nineteenth century that opposes much of modern medicine, instead believing that disease can be cured by prayer. As a result, several outbreaks have occurred in communities where this branch of Christianity is common. In 1985 an outbreak of measles occurred at Christian Science–affiliated Principia College, where approximately 113 of its 712 students were affected, including three deaths.[28] In the same year, an outbreak occurred at a Colorado camp, where 50 of its 110 campers developed measles.[29] In 1994 an outbreak began in Illinois, where 141 people with measles were associated with both a Christian Science boarding school and college.[30] Additionally, there have been outbreaks of polio and diphtheria associated with Christian Science communities in the past. This group permits vaccination when required by law[31] but does not believe it to be necessary.

The Church of Scientology is a religion founded in the 1950s by the science-fiction author L. Ron Hubbard. Scientologists publicly state, "Scientologists seek conventional medical treatment for illnesses and injuries. Scientologists use prescription drugs when physically ill and also rely on the advice and treatment of physicians." Scientologist Reverend John Carmichael has stated that there are no religious principles regarding vaccination within Scientology.[32] However because the church requires membership to learn certain nonpublic teachings, it is difficult to assess if the stated public position accurately reflects internal policies.

Jainism, a religion most common in India, has prohibitions against violence that typically include vegetarianism. The Jain religion doesn't prohibit vaccination (although it could be seen as harming microorganisms) because it is considered necessary to protect the health of individuals.

Hinduism, the third largest religion in the world, doesn't have prohibitions against vaccination. The use of cow parts, such as fetal bovine serum, in the production of certain vaccines has not become a major religious concern. Hinduism is comprised of many sects that may have differing rules and prohibitions. However, regions with large Hindu populations, such as India, have had successful immunization campaigns. India eliminated indigenous transmission of polio in 2011,[33] for example.

The Church of Jesus Christ of Latter-day Saints, a branch of Christianity previously commonly known as Mormonism,[34] has encouraged vaccination among its membership since at least 1978.[35] In 1985 the church issued an immunization reminder and referred to vaccination as an obligation.[36] The church has donated millions of dollars to immunization initiatives and in 2012 made immunization an official humanitarian initiative.[37]

Sikhism, the world's fifth largest organized religion, makes no prohibition against vaccination.

No Buddhist tradition opposes vaccination. Indeed, the Fourteenth Dalai Lama, Tenzin Gyatso, an important religious figure in some forms of Buddhism, himself vaccinated two children against polio on live television in 2010.

Neither of the two largest sects of Satanism, the Church of Satan and the Satanic Temple, oppose vaccination. The Church of Satan has an article on its website encouraging HPV vaccination. The Satanic Temple holds as a tenet, "One's body is inviolable, subject to one's own will alone." This may be interpreted as an opposition to mandatory vaccination;[38] however, vaccination is not mandatory in most jurisdictions, only required in order to attend school or day care.

Overall nearly every major religion in the world is either neutral to vaccination, holding no specific position on it, or actively encourages its members to become vaccinated. This hasn't stopped some parents from using religious exemptions as a means of avoiding vaccination, sometimes by lying about their religious beliefs or affiliation.[39] In 2002 a law was struck down in Arkansas that would have required parents to be affiliated with a specific organized religion to obtain a religious exemption, and states do not punish parents who falsify either their religious affiliation or the beliefs of their religion in order to avoid vaccination.[40]

These cases of seeking religious exemption for vaccination are largely a smokescreen that allows anti-vaccine activists to bypass normal vaccination requirements for children to attend schools or daycares. Rather than a true expression of religious faith, the use of religious vaccine exemptions is often an exploitation of the privileged status of religious faith in society.

Answering whether states should continue to allow religious exemptions is more difficult. In the United States, freedom of and from religion is a constitutional guarantee. However the government can place certain restrictions on religious practice. In the 1878 Supreme Court ruling *Reynolds v. United States*, the Supreme Court examined whether religious duty was a valid defense against a criminal indictment. Reynolds was a Mormon who had been convicted of bigamy, which he argued was his religious duty. The court considered the words of Thomas Jefferson in his letter to the Danbury Baptists—"Believing with you that religion is a matter which lies solely between Man & his God, that he owes account to none other for his faith or his worship, that the legitimate powers of government reach actions only, & not opinions"[41]—and found that "to permit this would be to make the professed doctrines of religious belief superior to the law of the land, and in effect to permit every citizen to become a law unto himself." This decision was reaffirmed in 1990 in *Employment Division v. Smith*. The case *Sherbet v. Verner* established the so-called Sherbert test, whereby government must demonstrate a "compelling state interest" to interfere with religious liberties.

Public health is such a compelling state interest. Freedom of religious belief is not the same as freedom of action premised on religious belief. The benefits of public health measures such as vaccination are strong. In the rare case that religious beliefs do conflict with vaccination, the state's interest in public health may outweigh religious privilege.

17 Big Pharma

The enemy is clearly delineated: he is a perfect model of malice, a kind of amoral superman—sinister, ubiquitous, powerful, cruel, sensual, luxury-loving. Unlike the rest of us, the enemy is not caught in the toils of the vast mechanism of history, himself a victim of his past, his desires, his limitations. He wills, indeed he manufactures, the mechanism of history, or tries to deflect the normal course of history in an evil way. He makes crises, starts runs on banks, causes depressions, manufactures disasters, and then enjoys and profits from the misery he has produced. The paranoid's interpretation of history is distinctly personal: decisive events are not taken as part of the stream of history, but as the consequences of someone's will.

—Richard Hofstadter, *The Paranoid Style in American Politics*[1]

A common theme in discussions of vaccines is the profit motive of pharmaceutical companies that manufacture them:[2] Big Pharma is lying to you. Big Pharma has bribed the government. Mandatory vaccination hands over new customers to Big Pharma. Media gets revenue from Big Pharma. They're lying to you too. Vaccine research isn't independent, so it's biased. Those who promote vaccination are shills for Big Pharma too! The payroll of Big Pharma is as endless and insidious as Monsanto's!

What is Big Pharma? How did it get this powerful? And are any of these claims true?

Big Pharma refers to dozens of companies, researchers, regulators, physicians, and scientists involved with the production of drugs and biologics, such as vaccines. Many big-pharma companies have given the public good reason to dislike and distrust them. One example involves the EpiPen, a device that automatically injects an appropriate dose of epinephrine to those suffering from life-threatening allergies. For them, this device is necessary and life-saving. It was developed by Sheldon Kaplan in the 1970s as the ComboPen,[3] which was to replace a previous autoinjector pen that had a stainless steel barrel. The EpiPen debuted in 1980 and was acquired by Mylan in 2007. Between 2007 and 2016, the price of an EpiPen rose more than 400 percent,[4] an increase possibly endangering the lives of those who could no longer afford them. The decision to raise the price of this device could not be justified as increased manufacturing or development costs because the device had been developed forty years prior and manufacturing costs had not increased 400 percent.

Another famous contemporary case came with "pharma bro" Martin Shkreli, who is now serving time in federal prison. Shkreli was CEO of Turing Pharmaceuticals, which acquired Daraprim, a medication for treating toxoplasmosis. Turing increased the price of Daraprim from $13.50 per pill to $750 per pill. Shkreli appeared to blame the media for the negative publicity surrounding the price hike. In 2015 he was arrested for financial fraud. In 2016 he was called to testify before Congress about the rate increases and refused to answer any question other than to give his name.

Indeed, at the start of 2019, more than one thousand drugs saw increases in price averaging well over inflation.[5] The often standard explanation that these increases reflect the cost of research ring hollow because many drugs were researched decades ago, and research costs are small compared to the money spent on marketing of drugs.[6] Another concern with the pharmaceutical companies is that their financial interests can lead them to bring unsafe products to market, Vioxx being a common example.

In 1999 the drug Vioxx was approved, manufactured by Merck. Vioxx was a nonsteroidal anti-inflammatory drug, which was used to treat arthritis and other diseases in over eighty million people. As early as 2001, an analysis indicated that Vioxx was leading to an increased risk of cardiovascular disease.[7] The authors suggested that the FDA mandate a trial to determine if Vioxx led to increased risk of cardiovascular disease, but the FDA did not. At the same time that studies began to show that Vioxx was leading to an increased risk of heart attack, Merck was spending more than $100 million per year on advertising the drug. In 2002 the FDA told Merck to include a notice of cardiovascular risks in the Vioxx package insert.[8] Merck was most likely aware of the cardiac risk profile of Vioxx,[9] but rather than endanger a drug that was bringing in billions of dollars in prescriptions, they continued to market it and provided materials to sales people, labeled "dodgeball Vioxx," for how to talk to customers about concerns over cardiovascular disease.[10] It later came out that one of the authors of studies showing the drug's efficacy had fabricated data in at least twenty-one studies.[11] In 2004 the drug was withdrawn following an internal study at Merck (ironically named APPROVe). A later FDA panel recommended bringing Vioxx back to market, given that the risk profile was likely not worse than those of some other pain killers.

These and other incidents have reinforced negative views of the pharmaceutical industry overall. A 2016 Gallup poll ranked the pharmaceutical industry as having a 51 percent negative and only 28 percent positive public perception,[12] just before the many news stories about the price of the EpiPen increasing. Many believe that there is a fundamental conflict between the motivations of corporations to make a profit and the needs of patients to receive safe and effective medications. This extends to criticism of the FDA's ties to the pharmaceutical industry, if not directly than through the ability of consultants to move freely between the public and private sectors. How might someone who was a part of the pharmaceutical industry, and almost certain to return to it as a consultant, possibly be objective while acting as a regulator at the FDA?

These ties between industry and the government agencies that regulate and approve drugs and vaccines produced by those industries create a public perception of rampant malfeasance. Until the 1962 amendment to the Federal Food, Drug, and Cosmetic Act, drug manufacturers were required to show only that drugs were safe, before bringing them to market. The 1962 act required manufacturers to show, as well, with "substantial" scientific evidence, that drugs were effective. Subsequent debates within the FDA, industry, and academic science shaped the way this law was interpreted. In special cases where there was already sufficient evidence of the safety and efficacy of a drug in many circumstances, a single, well-designed study was sometimes seen as adequate to expand a drug to other specific uses. An example of this would be a drug initially approved only for those between the ages fifteen and twenty-five being later approved for use by those up to the age of thirty. This flexibility was codified in the Modernization Act of 1997. Normally, however, independent substantiation of results is required, meaning that multiple studies, often with similar designs must be conducted. These studies must be in agreement, and even apparently well-designed multi-center trials may have subtle biases. Biologics, such as vaccines, have often been held to a higher standard than other drugs and are regulated under a different set of rules.

By contrast to the regulation of drugs and biologics, the regulation of products marketed as dietary supplements is extremely permissive. The Dietary Supplement Health and Education Act (DSHEA) of 1994 effectively exempts manufacturers of these substances from the need to demonstrate safety or efficacy. Manufacturers are required to label a product accurately, but under the DSHEA, the "United States shall bear the burden of proof on each element to show that a dietary supplement is adulterated." This means that the burden of proof lies not on the supplement maker to show that it is safe, as with vaccines or drugs, but on the FDA to show that it is unsafe—a more difficult and expensive task, given the vast variety of products marketed as supplements.

Between 2004 and 2012, half of the FDA-mandated recalls in the United States were supplements.[13] Often these recalls were for supplements' containing unlabeled active pharmaceutical products—meaning that the supplements were deemed unsafe because they might actually do something. However, I have been unable to find either complaints among anti-vaccine activists about the closeness of "Big Supplement" to legislators, about Big Supplement's safety issues and skirting of the laws, and about the secrecy of manufacturing processes by Big Supplement, or complaints about the ineffectiveness of nearly all supplements at solving the problems they are marketed as solving. Before the DSHEA legislation, the dietary-supplement industry was estimated to be about $4 billion per year. It is now predicted to surpass $200 billion per year by 2024.[14]

The legitimate reasons for people's dislike of pharmaceutical companies are often muddied by conspiracy theories. Like many conspiracy theories, they involve a belief that a small number of people are working in secret against the public good, a belief that most people are unaware of what's really happening and only conspiracy theorists know the truth, and a set of way of handling evidence that spins disconfirmatory evidence into conspiracy beliefs.[15] The conflicting, complex, and shifting motivations and incentives of lobbyists, physicians, scientists, regulators, and politicians are simplified to villainous greed. Although it's tempting to dismiss such conspiracies outright because conspiracy theorists tend to be wrong about everything, there have historically been actual conspiracies. So it is worthwhile both to address why people believe in conspiracy theories, even after the absence of confirmatory evidence becomes overwhelming, and to examine the evidence put forward for those conspiracy theories in particular.

One explanation for such conspiracy-minded behavior is an overabundance of fundamental attribution bias (FAB).[16] FAB is a phenomenon where people are willing to attribute to themselves a complex set of motivations and situational reasons for behavior, and attribute the same behavior in others to fundamental characteristics of those people. An example would be saying, "Steve is bad at managing his finances," rather than "Steve made several bad investments because he got bad advice." Or saying, "Lucy is a poor driver," rather than "Lucy was in a rush that day because her spouse was in labor at the hospital." This kind of bias applies to pharmaceutical companies because when something goes poorly, such as the recall of Vioxx, it is easy to attribute the negative behavior to fundamental traits of the company, rather than to the individual circumstances of that case. Did the Merck executives know for certain that Vioxx could cause heart attacks and suppress the information to continue making a profit? Or did they err because they based their decision on the data available to them and simply made a mistake? However, as tempting as this explanation may be, it would require that Big Pharma conspiracists were overall more prone to FAB than were nonconspiracists—a hypothesis that lacks strong evidence either way.[17]

Another explanation for conspiracy-minded thinking is that those feeling they lack control in their lives seek frameworks of belief that are coherent and internally resilient to outside challenges. To a conspiracist, someone debunking Big Pharma as conspiracy theory must a part of the conspiracy.[18] In a 2008 report, J. A. Whitson and A. D. Galinsky showed that participants who felt they lacked control were more likely to perceive a conspiracy.[19] In that way the conspiracy theory is less likely to be accurate but is protected from challenge. Those who believe in conspiracy theories are more susceptible to conjunction errors.[20] Those are mistakes in thinking in which it is believed that multiple events are more probable than are those events on their own.[21] Conspiracy believers are also likely to attribute intent where none exists.[22]

The philosopher of science Karl Popper wrote about conspiracies theories in his essay "The Conspiracy Theory of Society," comparing conspiracy belief to theistic religious belief. While in a religious belief, stochastic phenomena, such as the weather, are attributed to supernatural intervention by gods, in conspiracy theories, the stochastic outcomes of complex systems are attributed to sinister and powerful groups and individuals.[23] Although Popper acknowledged that conspiracies exist, he pointed out that human designs rarely ever go according to plan. Try as we might to take actions that only have intended consequences, every action has unintended consequences as well. So trying to understand society from a model in which every event was intended to occur by some person or group misses the stochastic nature of many events.

One critic of Popper's view of conspiracies, Charles Pigden, argued that conspiracy theories weren't superstitious at all, but represented an accurate view of history.[24] In this model conspiracies can be a valid explanation for some of the phenomena in history, but not *all* phenomena. There are numerous examples of real conspiracies in history, such as the Watergate scandal, and we are only aware of them because they were unsuccessful. In this model it is still important to separate signal from noise. Conspiracy theorists are often talking about the Popperian style of conspiracy, so real-life conspiracies may only serve to demonstrate how difficult it is to actually carry out such malfeasance without it eventually coming to light.

In *The Paranoid Style in American Politics*, Richard Hofstadter suggested that those with conspiracy beliefs are prone to collect evidence, not to determine the truth, but to protect themselves from it. It is an acknowledged truth of pharmacology that all drugs have side effects, and that sometimes these side effects are painful, unpleasant, or deadly. The scientist studying pharmacology examines the evidence for these side effects, which is recorded, weighed against the effects of the disease being treated and the effectiveness of the treatment, and sometimes accepted as a part of an aggregate good that offering a treatment provides. To a conspiracist, these side effects, or the occasional failure of a treatment to work, provide evidence that confirms what they already knew, that Big Pharma is a sinister entity, manipulating the government, and spreading disease.[25] After all, when someone comes down with an untreatable disease, it is natural to ask, *Cui bono*? Who benefits? Pharmaceutical companies become a tangible target for those seeking an enemy to rally against.

The market forces that drive pharmaceutical companies don't always favor the production of drugs that consumers need. Research into new antibiotics has slowed to a near stall because of the high cost of bringing new drugs to market, and the low economic returns on antibiotics that are only prescribed for short courses.[26] Likewise vaccines, which are often inexpensive, yield comparatively little profit for pharmaceutical companies. Out of nearly $1 trillion in annual revenues,[27] only about $20 billion are revenues from vaccines,[28] likely the net profit from these vaccines is much less when costs of production, research, taxes, and so forth are taken into account. These profits, are small compared to the potential profits from sales of drugs to treat someone hospitalized for a preventable disease.

Regardless of the morality of drug-pricing schemes, and dismissing for a moment the Popperian kind of conspiracy where a small secret group is operating to make decisions that impact the entire drug industry, does a profit motive invalidate the safety or efficacy of vaccines? There are, in fact, biases in the publication of results by manufacturers. For example, in manufacturer-supported trials, publication is far more likely to show positive results than it is in publicly funded trials. Studies of nonsteroidal anti-inflammatory drugs showed almost exclusively that publications supported greater or equal efficacy and safety than for comparison drugs.[29] Drug studies funded by manufacturers and published in proceedings of symposia are far more likely to show a positive result for the drug of interest than are publicly funded studies (98 percent vs. 79 percent).[30] However, although there is less likelihood that pharmaceutical companies will publish a negative result, the results of individual studies are less likely to show bias.[31]

It's important to understand how this bias works. Industry funding affects research results in two ways: first, by violations of the "uncertainty principle," that is, the principle that clinical trials should only be conducted when there is uncertainty as to the effectiveness of a treatment.[32] A trial should select a control treatment for which the outcome is uncertain, rather than one that is not comparable. This means that a new drug should be compared to the current standard drug on the market and not to a placebo. The second means by which industry funding influences research is called publication bias, or the file-drawer effect. Businesses are less likely than nonprofits are to publish discouraging results. This may be the result of deliberately deciding not to publish, ending a trial early that might produce negative results, or selecting trials to perform that already have a high likelihood of producing positive results. These are serious sources of bias that influence the scientific record, but importantly they lack several of the features of conspiracy theories.

The conspiracy model usually has Big Pharma deliberately falsifying studies in order to sell products. The truth is far more mundane. Although the profit motive produces biases, those biases don't much affect the results of individual studies. Moreover, often the initial development of drugs and vaccines are publicly funded through research grants from the National Institutes of Health. The perverse incentives created by the profit motive of the pharmaceutical industry are overridden by sound science and adequate regulation.

Once again a comparison to the unregulated supplement industry is apt. If the pharmaceutical industry operated the same way that the dietary supplement industry does, *Cui bono?* would be a more appropriate question. Though dietary supplements do have important health uses, such as folate during pregnancy, these are a tiny fraction of the dietary supplements marketed, the majority of which are not based on evidence. Many contain substances other than those on the label, which are sometimes toxic. All in the name of profit. The industry surrounding supplements is exactly what anti-vaccine advocates fear about vaccines: unregulated, unsafe, and ineffective. By comparison, the testing required to bring a vaccine to market ensures a high likelihood of safety and efficacy.

An attitude that denies vaccine safety and efficacy based on the profit motives of the companies that produce them is also inconsistent with the use of other less maligned medicines. Big Pharma produces antibiotics, insulin, epinephrine, steroids to prevent anaphylaxis, and every other life-saving medication. Yet very few people refuse medical treatment overall, and those who do report other reasons, such as low perceived need, high cost, poor insurance, or, most often, distrust of physicians.[33]

Few entities are well funded enough and motivated to do the kinds of expenditures that are required to develop new vaccines. Governmental agencies, nonprofits, and corporations can all to some degrees fill those roles, but currently the majority of new drugs are brought to market by large corporations, following basic development conducted with grants from the federal government. Nonprofit organizations also offer grants, and many corporations conduct research in-house. Ownership of the tangible products of this research is a question still debated. Those who conducted government-funded research are often required to make their findings publicly available. However, meeting the technical and safety requirements to produce a vaccine is a large undertaking. Not only must vaccines be produced under sterile conditions and in a high quality; they must also be tested; the steps in production audited; the equipment used, recalibrated cleaned, and maintained on a schedule; and meticulous records kept.

The goalposts to determine that a vaccine is safe are as high or higher than they are for other kinds of drugs. Currently, in the United States, vaccines are evaluated by the Center for Biologics Evaluation and Research (CBER) at the FDA. The development of government agencies to regulate the safety of biologics followed the "horse named Jim" scandal. In the nineteenth century, diphtheria epidemics were common. The disease affected mainly children and had a high mortality rate. The bacterium that causes diphtheria was first cultured in 1884.[34] It was discovered that the bacterium produced a toxin and that animals injected with the toxin produced a substance in their blood that could help treat diphtheria. Within a decade factories were established to produce antitoxin.

In 1901 a horse (named Jim) was bled to produce antitoxin, and two days later was euthanized due to a tetanus infection. The blood was ordered to be destroyed, but within weeks at least thirteen children died of tetanus infections.[35] The deaths received significant publicity and fearful parents refused antitoxin treatment, their refusal increasing the number of deaths due to diphtheria. This and other incidents, such as a series of eight deaths from contaminated smallpox vaccine, lead to the Biologics Control Act in 1902.

The Biologics Control Act established a board, including the surgeons general of the army, the navy, and the Marine Hospital Service, to oversee production of antitoxins and vaccines. Labs producing vaccines could be inspected at random; labeling requirements were instituted; and the board was given the power to issue or revoke licenses to produce vaccines. This was one of the first cases of government oversight of the safety of vaccine production and created the precedent that the federal government would oversee vaccine safety going forward, Ultimately it led to the creation of the FDA.

The exact mission and scope of what is now CBER has changed over time; however, currently it is tasked with ensuring the safety of vaccines in the United States. This includes maintaining VAERs and licensing manufacturers. Within CBER is the Vaccines and Related Biological Products Advisory Committee (VRBPAC), tasked with reviewing and evaluating data concerning the safety, effectiveness, and appropriate use of vaccines and biological products intended for use in the prevention, treatment, or diagnosis of human diseases."[36] This committee is composed of fifteen members chosen for their qualifications, such as expertise in clinical fields and experience in "interpreting complex data." Most members have a doctorate in medicine or philosophy in a related field. Detailed reporting of potential (perceived or real) conflicts of interest, such as financial interests in companies, employment, or research grants, is required.[37]

Research starts in a preclinical phase with scientists who test vaccine candidates. Various types of vaccine might be developed, including live-attenuated virus, inactivated (dead) virus, recombinant/subunit/polysaccharide/conjugate vaccines, or toxoid vaccines.[38] Next, when possible, animal trials are completed. Animals are used as what scientists call "model organisms," or organisms with biological similarities to humans. A drug or vaccine that kills mice or makes them sick, for example, won't be used in humans because of the risk that it may also harm humans. If the disease being vaccinated against is one that infects a model organism, it may also be possible to test if the candidate vaccine is able to prevent disease in that organism.

If a candidate vaccine has been shown to be safe in model organisms, it will usually be tested in humans for safety. Typically the first phase involves this safety testing. The second phase, involving more participants, determines the appropriate dose. And finally phase-three clinical trials are the most comprehensive, involving thousands of people. Only a small fraction of potential drugs or vaccines make it to the stage of clinical trials. The FDA reviews the data produced by trials as they go on and may stop trials at any point if they appear to be unsafe or ineffective. The success rate for treatments that make it to the clinical-trial phase are very low, only a little more than 10 percent.[39] Many times more are tested or examined in labs, but the evidence is never sufficient to move them to the stage of clinical trials. The clinical trial process is expensive and difficult to navigate, but for good reason—to ensure that the drugs and vaccines delivered in health care are safe, effective, and of high quality. Since 1997, an average of $1.4 billion was spent each year on vaccine research and development, 46 percent from vaccine sales, 36 percent from taxes, and 18 percent from risk capital.[40]

Many of the major problems with the pharmaceutical industry, and the public-private partnership that produces and tests new drugs, can be fixed. Journal editors have the opportunity to give space to more publications with negative results. Companies either should (or should be required to) make all trial data public, regardless of their results. Companies spend more on the marketing of drugs than they do on research, and some of that research is itself intended to market drugs. These are problems that can be solved through regulation, but in no way mean that vaccines are unsafe, or do not protect against disease.

The year 2018 saw a 30 percent increase in measles cases world-wide,[1] from nineteen cases per million to twenty-five cases per million, attributed by health professionals to the effects of the anti-vaccine movement.[2] That same year also saw over one hundred thousand measles-related deaths worldwide. While 95 percent coverage is believed to be required to prevent outbreaks, global coverage has stalled at 85 percent and is lower in some regions. Figure 18.1 shows how measles cases in 2018 and early 2019 have increased compared with previous years.

Losses such as these should also be considered in the context of gains. More children than ever received the DTP vaccine in 2017; the number of undervaccinated children in the world has decreased in the last decade; and hundreds of thousands to millions of lives have been saved by vaccination programs. Since 2010 the percentage of children receiving the second dose of the measles vaccine has risen from 39 percent to 67 percent in 2017. Although polio was targeted for elimination in 2015, and still had three dozen new wild cases in 2018 and is unlikely to be fully eliminated by 2020, it is still nearing elimination.

In November 2018 an outbreak of chickenpox, affecting thirty-six students, occurred in North Carolina at a Waldorf

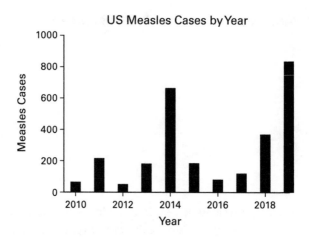

Figure 18.1
The return of measles to the United States: the year 2019 saw a measles outbreak in the United States, with more cases than in previous years, which has to be partially attributed to the anti-vaccine movement. Data from the CDC, www.cdc.gov/measles/cases-outbreaks.html.

School. This school had one of the lowest vaccination rates in the state, with nineteen of twenty-eight students in the kindergarten class having received religious vaccine exemptions.[3] Waldorf schools often have concentrations of undervaccinated children. In 2015 Austin Waldorf School in Travis County, Texas, had the second highest exemption rate in Texas at 48 percent.[4] Lake Champlain Waldorf School in Vermont had only a 50 percent vaccination rate.[5] A Belmont Heights, California, Waldorf School had only 20 percent of its students up to date with vaccinations.[6] And in the Seattle school district, a Waldorf School had the highest vaccine-exemption rate, 40 percent.[7]

Rockland County, New York, is experiencing an ongoing measles outbreak with hundreds of cases so far (figure 18.2),[8]

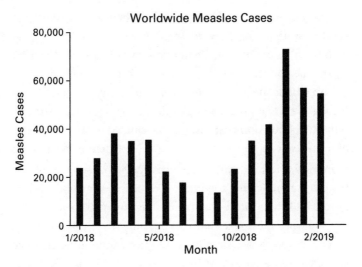

Figure 18.2
The 2018 and 2019 measles outbreaks: Worldwide measles cases increased in 2019 compared with 2018, likely partially due to the effect of the anti-vaccine movement. Data from the WHO.

the outbreak was traced to an unvaccinated child who had traveled to Israel where more than 1,300 measles cases occurred in 2018.[9] In Europe more than 41,000 people were infected with measles in the first half of 2018.[10] The hardest hit country was Ukraine, with over 20,000 cases. In February 2019 a measles outbreak occurred in Clark County, Washington, where a medical emergency was declared after 49 cases occurred. In Clark County the measles-vaccination rate was only 78 percent.[11] This has led to a bipartisan effort in the Washington legislature to eliminate personal and philosophical exemptions in that state. Recently several states, including Maine and Washington, have passed legislation making it more difficult to obtain exemptions.

Outbreaks are most likely to occur when vaccination levels fall below that necessary for herd immunity. When enough members of a population are immune to a disease, the probability of a person who is not immune coming into contact with a person who is infectious goes down. Immunity can be acquired through vaccination or through infection and survival. The fraction of a population that must be vaccinated to stop the spread of a disease can be calculated as $V_c = \frac{q_c}{E}$, where q_c is the herd-immunity threshold, and R_0 is the basic reproductive number of the disease, indicating the number of people someone with the disease is likely to infect. If a vaccine is less than 100 percent effective, then we must take that into account when calculating the vaccine coverage necessary to achieve herd immunity. This necessary vaccine coverage, V_c, can be calculated as $V_c = \frac{q_c}{E}$, where E is the effectiveness of the vaccine. The measles vaccine is 97 percent effective but the R_0 of measles is very high. The estimate for the R_0 of measles is often cited as 12 to 18, but estimates are higher than this.[12] Regardless, this means that the vaccine coverage necessary to protect a population from measles ranges from 95 percent to 98 percent.

Measles vaccine coverage remains steady at 85 percent worldwide, which is far from achieving the goal of immunization levels at or above the critical threshold for herd immunity, and is responsible for the 30 percent spike in measles in 2018. Even the 91 percent coverage in the United States is inadequate to prevent the spread of measles in the population. Some cannot afford or access health care, but those who can and choose not to contribute to the population's immunity increase its susceptibility to outbreaks. Opposition to vaccination contributes to these numbers. Moreover, these estimates assume a homogenous population. Enclaves such as Waldorf schools can harbor rates of vaccine coverage far lower even than the population average and thus are particularly dangerous for the immune compromised and others with legitimate medical reasons for which they cannot be vaccinated.

In 2017–2018 the influenza season was at high severity across all age groups. According to the CDC, 185 children died from influenza.[13] There were over 80,000 flu-related deaths in the United States, making it the most deadly flu season in a decade.[14]

Meanwhile, anti-vaccine activists have continued to try new strategies. In September the organization Learn the Risk put up a billboard in Kansas City with the words "As a nurse I was never taught vaccines can kill until my son was a victim."[15] In August 2018 an anti-vaccine nurse made news when she used social media to discuss a measles patient under her care, stating that seeing the symptoms helped her to understand why people vaccinate but that she would continue to oppose vaccination. She was subsequently fired from Texas Children's Hospital for revealing confidential patient information online.[16] Rallies have been held by anti-vaccine activists in some of the areas hardest hit by the 2019 measles outbreak.

In Italy the governing party of the League and the Five Star Movement were elected promising to oppose mandatory vaccination. Italy's health minister allowed parents to self-certify that their children had been vaccinated. The Italian parliament has stated that proof of vaccination has only been delayed.[17] In September 2018 the coalition scrapped its vaccination reforms. As the European measles outbreak continued into November 2018, the Italian coalition government's health ministry called for widespread vaccination against measles.[18] Adding to this confusion, in early December, the health minister fired the

commission of health experts that in November had recommended widespread vaccination.[19]

In Germany in 2019, there was one of the highest rates of
measles in Europe with more than six hundred cases. Subsequently, the German government has made plans to institute
significant fines for parents who do not vaccinate.[20] These plans
are contingent on action by the German parliament.

The election of explicitly anti-vaccination political parties in
Italy may be unprecedented in an explicitly anti-vaccine political party coming to power, an inversion of the usual relationship
between establishment health authorities and antiestablishment
anti-vaccine activists, and is particularly ill-timed given the current outbreak of measles.

In twelve of eighteen US states that track nonmedical vaccine exemptions (NMEs) rates of NMEs rose in 2018, part of an
overall upward trend since at least 2009;[21] however, in several
states the rise in NMEs in the early half of the decade has leveled
off. This is despite educational programs in some states requiring parents to watch videos or complete an educational module
before obtaining an NME.

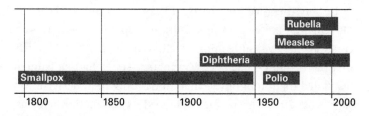

Figure 18.3
Time from the introduction or discovery of a vaccine against a variety of
infectious diseases to the last endemic case of that disease in the United
States.

Recent data has also suggested a change in the political ideology of anti-vaccine activists. A 2018 internet survey including questions about political polarization and intent to vaccinate found a weak correlation between conservative beliefs and lack of intent to vaccinate.[22] This contrasts with prior studies that have shown no link between political affiliation and intent to vaccinate.

On balance, the present state of public health efforts and anti–public health efforts is a mix of both good and bad news. Vaccine coverage continues to increase, but not fast enough to prevent outbreaks of measles. Nonmedical exemptions rose but plateaued, and anti-vaccine activists have continued to invent new ways to prevent immunization, frighten the public, and push for bad legislation.

19   Vaccine Advocates

Then assembles youth's fairest flower to see your play, and listens to the revelation. Then every gentle mind sucks melancholy nourishment for itself from out your work; then one while this, and one while that, is stirred up; each one sees what he carries in his heart.

—Johann Wolfgang von Goethe, *Faust*, part 1

As anti-vaccine activists have opposed vaccination, a variety of institutions, groups, and individuals have chosen to become advocates for vaccination. These vaccine advocates each have unique motivations, and each have used a variety of strategies with various degrees of effectiveness. Future effectiveness of vaccine advocates will benefit from attention to those strategies that have been shown to increase a person's likelihood to vaccinate, and to avoid those that result in backfire effects, or fruitless, emotionally charged arguments.

Several studies have addressed methods of promoting vaccination, with mixed results. Nyan and colleagues found that the use of a dramatic narrative about a sick child who was not vaccinated, or images of children suffering from vaccine-preventable illness, actually decreased the desire of parents to vaccinate their children. Textual information from the CDC showing that there was no vaccine-autism link reduced misconception about that proposed link but did not increase intent to vaccinate.[1] This suggests that inventions focused on correcting misconceptions about vaccines, raising concerns about communicable diseases, or simply filling an information deficit may be ineffective.

However, other methods have been successful in increasing intent to vaccinate. Providing an HPV fact sheet was enough to increase intent to vaccinate from 49 percent to 70 percent in one group.[2] Parents receiving vaccine information pamphlets had greater intent to vaccinate (76 percent versus 38 percent) and were less likely to turn to nonmedical sources of information.[3] An informational pamphlet increases parents' intent to vaccinate their daughters about HPV.[4] Graphical presentation has also been shown to be effective in increasing intent to vaccinate,[5] and a *radionovela*[6] has been shown to be an effective, culturally tailored means of providing information about HPV vaccination.[7] Web-based decision aids have also been effectively used to increase intent to vaccinate with MMR. A marketing campaign developed a set of materials based on interviews with local parents to determine their concerns, and distributed brochures and fliers in the offices of health-care providers and heavily frequented community centers, such as pharmacies and grocery stores. Eighty-two percent of targeted respondents had seen the materials, and there was a modest 2 percent increase in vaccination rates in studied counties in the following months.[8] In Pakistan, meetings with community members to factually discuss vaccination with encouragement to spread those discussions to the community were successful in increasing the odds of measles and DPT vaccination.[9] A community in Australia implemented a campaign, "I Immunise," specifically targeting a community with high vaccine hesitancy by addressing community values and identity. This was based on the premise that letting people know what others in their community are doing can promote prosocial behavior.[10] The campaign improved vaccine attitudes for 77 percent of respondents but further polarized those who responded negatively.[11] A Washington State program, the Immunity Community, implemented a social-marketing training program to train community members as "vaccine advocates" who provide factual information to other members of the community. Targeted communities saw significant improvements in vaccine hesitancy.[12] These results suggest two broadly defined methods as being effective in increasing intent to vaccinate: providing factual information about vaccines[13] and providing community- and identity-centered messaging about vaccines.

While many organizations and individuals make use of these factual and community strategies for vaccine advocacy, there is also a *reactive* strategy used in a great deal of science communication related to vaccines. This strategy involves the social shaming of anti-vaccine activists through sharing of memes, online mockery, and long-winded rebuttals to anti-vaccine messaging and media (see chapter 14). While these strategies are enjoyable, funny, or make us feel good in relation to targets within the anti-vaccine movement, they are not particularly evidence based and in some cases may do more harm than good. Reactive approaches carry with them the possibility of further polarizing the vaccine hesitant and turning them into anti-vaccine activists.

A reactive strategy can be prone to what's known as the backfire effect, which occurs when someone with a prior set of beliefs is exposed to new, contradictory information. Something funny happens: they become more set in their original belief, or at least they hold on to their favored but erroneous views. For example, those who were predisposed to support the US invasion of Iraq became more confident in their position after being corrected about their mistaken belief that Iraq had possessed weapons of mass destruction.[14] Likewise, when liberals were corrected in the belief that President George W. Bush had banned stem-cell research, the effect of the correction was similar to the effect experienced by conservatives corrected about WMDs in Iraq. Those who were supporters of vice presidential candidate Sarah Palin were more likely to believe that the Affordable Care Act would result in death panels, when shown a correction.[15] Showing parents information refuting a link between MMR vaccine and autism decreases their intent to vaccinate their children.[16] Subsequent studies of the backfire effect have not been able to replicate the increased entrenchedness of the views studied, but have been able to replicate the continued belief in erroneous information.

Engaging directly in reactive corrections on the internet also quickly runs into the problem of the so-called Gish Gallop. The Gish Gallop is named for the creationist Duane Gish, who was known for producing a series of weak arguments and false statements in rapid succession. When opponents responded, they would be left unable to address every point because it can take longer to refute every point than was allotted for rebuttal. An example run into frequently is "200 evidence-based reasons NOT to Vaccinate," a long list of cherry-picked article titles circulated to frighten readers into not vaccinating. Because the list is presented without the context of a broader view of the field, or professional interpretation, refuting each reason becomes a long, drawn-out, tedious exercise, or else the anti-vaccine activist declares victory.

Many public health institutions have taken a more measured approach. In the United States, federal agencies have chosen to take a generally *factual* strategy. The CDC provides fact sheets on its website with information about the contents of vaccines and how they are tested and evaluated. However, to find this information you must be interested enough to go looking for it. A vaccine denialist who is skeptical of government, or more interested in personal stories than dry fact sheets, may skip over CDC webpages.

The difficulty in implementing a factual strategy is compounded by the difficulty in demarking evidence-based information from counterfactual writing that takes a similar format. A parent searching for information on vaccination will not necessarily be first directed to trustworthy sources. A search on Amazon's online shopping portal makes no distinction between anti-vaccine books and reliable sources of information.[17] Factual information presented without the PR campaign of counterfactual information can become lost or more difficult to access.

Often, approaches to science communication involve creating a layer of interpretation, or misinterpretation, between scientists and the public. A handful of academics defy these norms and speak publicly on behalf of public health efforts. Among them, Peter Hotez, David Gorski, Steven Novella, and Paul Offit, coinventor of the rotavirus vaccine RotaTeq, and others have spoken out against anti-vaccine misinformation. Other academic scientists and physicians may not speak out, but by virtue of our profession, we each have a platform from which to speak. If not to tens of thousands of people, then at least to our friends and neighbors. Science communication can be democratized so that all scientists are communicators speaking directly to their communities.

If religious leaders should be criticized when they promote vaccine denial, then they should also be praised in the situations where a community vaccine-advocacy approach has worked. Religion is a large part of many people's lives and in many cases serves as a hub of community activity. This gives religious leaders an opportunity to participate in public health efforts by spreading good information.

Likewise, just as social media can be used by anti-vaccine activists to spread misinformation, it has the same potential to spread good information. Facebook and Twitter users can post photographs of themselves getting the flu shot—showing their followers what they are doing—as was done for the Australian "I Immunize" campaign. Parents can show their community members photographs of themselves getting their children vaccinated. Using a factual approach, social-media users can share fact sheets during flu season, as well as positive factual information about vaccines.

Some have managed to develop large online followings with pro-vaccine messaging. Stephan Neidenbach, a teacher at a public middle school, runs the group We Love GMOs and Vaccines, which has over 190,000 followers on Facebook. Other Facebook groups with large followings include Refutations to Anti-vaccine Memes, with 250,000 followers; The REAL Truth about Vaccines, with 1,600 followers; and Pro-vaccine Memes in the Style of Anti-vaccine Memes, with 2,800 followers. Although groups such as these can be prone to a reactive style of vaccine advocacy, they can still serve as an important counterpoint to anti-vaccine rhetoric that exists and spreads in the same medium.

Following the Disneyland measles outbreak, Vaccinate California, a parent advocacy group was formed by Leah Russin, a lawyer; Hannah Henry, a designer and educator; Renee Diresta; and Jennifer Wonnacott.[18] After SB-277 was introduced by senators Richard Pan and Ben Allen,[19] Vaccinate California gathered signatures for petitions, testified in the state legislature, and helped rally public support for the bill.

Richard Pan, trained as a pediatrician, first proposed vaccine legislation in the California assembly in 2012 with AB-2109, which required that parents seeking personal-belief exemptions provide evidence that a health-care provider had provided council to the parent about the health benefits and risks of vaccines.[20]

Leah Russin, one of the founders of Vaccinate California, related in an interview how she came to be involved with vaccine advocacy. During the 2014 Disneyland outbreak, she attended classes at a local family center with her fourteen-month-old child. A woman brought in her child who had not been vaccinated, and even though the child's older sibling had survived pertussis, she insisted that whooping cough was "no big deal." Russin was horrified that other families' children were being exposed to a preventable disease in an outbreak year. The family center had been a safe place to bring her child, but finding an unvaccinated child was like finding a "serpent in Eden." She was furious that good parents had been misled by people with a profit motive to "sell books or essential oils." She felt that although there are many parenting choices such as formula versus breastfeeding and when to introduce solids, those only affect your own family. Because vaccination affects the community, it should be "separate and apart from questions of what kind of parent should I be?"

Russin continued to research and discovered that some of the preschools in her area had allowed in children with personal-belief exemptions. She was shocked, living next to Stanford University, that people were "buying into nonsense." She decided that she needed to work to fix this problem in order to protect her kids. A lawyer who had worked in government, she knew a

number of politicians around California. She asked state senator
Dr. Richard Pan why he had only required that parents seeking
a personal-belief exemption be counseled by a health-care provider, rather than ban personal-belief exemptions outright. He
told her that in 2012 he had not had access to parent-advocates.
He had the support of health-care providers, but it was politi-
cally difficult to pass legislation in which the opposition were
parent groups.

Vaccinate California was founded as a parent group by Russin and others to support legislation to eliminate personal-belief
exemptions. This legislation came in the form of SB-277. SB-277
prevented the admission of students to elementary schools, secondary schools, and day care centers who had not been fully
immunized for a number of diseases.[21] Ultimately legislators and
advocates were successful, and SB-277 was signed into law in
2015. Effectively, SB-277 eliminated personal-belief exemptions
in California. The state's vaccination rates increased in the following years; however, they plateaued below 95 percent. Russin believes that this is due to loopholes surrounding medical
exemptions and unscrupulous physicians selling medical exemptions as a "side hustle." Parents could communicate online and
in social circles the names of physicians willing to provide such
exemptions. This could lead to local clusters of unvaccinated
children. In California there is no way to invalidate an unjusti-
fied exemption.

In 2019 SB-276 was introduced to address these loopholes.
SB-276 would mean that a medical exemption would require an
application to the state department of public health. The department would consider an application on the basis of medical
justification and supporting data. Absent such justification the
exemption would be denied with the possibility for appeal. At

the initial hearing for SB-276, in late April 2019, a large number of anti-vaccine activists appeared to speak against the bill. However, it passed committee and will move on to the appropriations committee. In September 2019 an anti-vaccine protestor disrupted a California State Senate hearing by using a menstrual cup to splash blood on several lawmakers.[22]

Russin advises those hoping to copy Vaccinate California's success to first identify a state legislator willing to take on passing legislation. Next, she advises pro-vaccine advocates to find or build a coalition of pro-vaccine groups that don't just include physicians. Physicians are expected to favor vaccination. So school nurses and PTA members are more compelling, especially when backed by every medical association in the state. Finally, she advises pro-vaccine advocates to find both parents and compelling stories. A compelling story is more likely to be shared on social media. Journalists are more likely to be interested in a personal story than in yet another study showing that MMR doesn't cause autism, and senators will find it hard to vote against legislation in the face of a sick kid. However, Russin warns potential pro-vaccine activists about the psychological toll that pro-vaccine work can take. During her work with Vaccinate California she was doxed.[23] Anti-vaccine activists showed up to picket her home. Someone spoofed a police-department email address and send her an email saying that they know who she is and that no one would respond if she made a 911 call. Richard Pan was able to stay stoic as anti-vaccine activists brought forth children they claimed were "vaccine injured" and begged him not to pass SB-276. Moreover, the most tempting form of activism, debating anti-vaccine activists online, one on one, is in her view ineffective and only leads to pro-vaccine activists burning themselves out. Debating anti-vaccine activists forces them to articulate their view and, in doing so, makes them more entrenched in it. Better, in Russin's view, is to publicly be a good parent and model for others that good parenting includes vaccinating one's own children.

Vaccination occupies a unique space as one of the most effective technologies ever developed to fight disease, as well as the only technology to ever eliminate a disease entirely. Vaccination conveys both individual and collective benefits, and carries very modest individual and collective risks. Individuals assessing those benefits and risks for themselves and their children deserve to do so with the best possible information available. Each person reading this book has a voice that can be used to help spread good information, to help set a good example for their friends and neighbors, and to help make the world a healthier place.

20 Who Are They?

To understand the anti-vaccine movement, we also need to understand its composition. Are some groups more likely to be vaccine hesitant than others? A distinction should be made between anti-vaccine activists who devote significant time and resources to spreading misinformation and communicating with other anti-vaccine activists and the merely vaccine-hesitant. The vaccine hesitant may have heard some negative things about vaccines, but they have not entirely made up their minds. Another distinction should be made for the undervaccinated because there are reasons a child may not be vaccinated other than opposition to vaccines.

A 2017 study looked at who made up anti-vaccine activists. Sociologists Naomi Smith and Tim Graham studied six large anti-vaccine groups on Facebook. Because the Facebook application programming interface does not provide demographic data, genders were estimated based on user's given names.[1] Smith and Graham found that on average the ratio of men to women users was 1:3 and that the gender ratio was even more skewed for the most active users in these groups.[2] Analysis of common topics discussed within these groups showed that common themes were activism, governance, media/censorship/cover up, vaccination as genocide, Zika virus/Gates Foundation, moral transgressions, vaccine injury, food as medicine, and chemtrail/ agriculture. These topics suggested that anti-vaccine activists view vaccination as a kind of institutional oppression and use Facebook to express moral outrage at the conspiracy of media and powerful interests that perpetuate vaccination.

A 2015 pew survey looking at the vaccine hesitant suggested, however, that men were slightly more likely than women to say they believe that the MMR vaccine is unsafe (11 percent versus 8 percent).[3] The survey also found similar rates of doubt for Republicans, Democrats, and Independents,[4] but higher rates for those with a less than high school education. If the general population of those with vaccine doubt has more men than women, why are the most active anti-vaccine activists women? One would expect that the leadership of anti-vaccine activists might reflect the composition of the vaccine hesitant.

The most likely explanation for this disparity I can find is that in the United States women still spend more time on childcare than men do,[5] and according to the US Department of Labor, "Mothers make approximately 80 percent of health care decisions for their children."[6] Mothers, being more involved in health decisions for children, might be more likely to seek out information from anti-vaccine sources.

Geographic distribution of anti-vaccination rhetoric is not uniform. An analysis of anti-vaccine tweets was able to find demographic characteristics that explained some of the geographic clustering of the tweets. California, Connecticut, Massachusetts, New York, and Pennsylvania had a higher volume of anti-vaccine tweets than you would expect based solely on population. Tweets were associated with "women who recently gave birth, households with high income levels, men aged 40 to 44, and men with minimal college education."[7]

The undervaccinated do not necessarily represent the same population as anti-vaccine activists. According to a 2004 study, undervaccinated children "tended to be black, to have a younger mother who was not married and did not have a college degree, to live in a household near the poverty level, and to live in a central city," while unvaccinated children "tended to be white, to have a mother who was married and had a college degree, to live in a household with an annual income exceeding 75,000 dollars, and to have parents who expressed concerns regarding the safety of vaccines and indicated that medical doctors have little influence over vaccination decisions for their children."[8] Undervaccinated children are likely to be children whose parents want them to receive health care but cannot afford it, whereas unvaccinated children are likely to be children of parents with vaccine doubt. Indeed, the strongest predictors of vaccine exemptions in California are median household income, higher percentage of white race in the population, and private schools.[9]

These differences underline the role of race and class privilege in the anti-vaccine movement. By its nature vaccination requires the participation of the majority to protect those in the minority who cannot be vaccinated for medical reasons or who do not have access to medical care. Those with access to medical care must be vaccinated for those without access to medical care to be protected or for those with medical conditions that make them unable to receive vaccines to be protected.

Other than wealth, race, and gender, what distinguishes those who do not vaccinate their children from those who do? They tend to have a lower level of trust in health-care professionals, a lower level of trust in government, a concern that a child's immune system could be "weakened" by too many immunizations, a belief that immunization requirements abridged freedom of choice and that parents know what's best for their own children, a greater level of trust in alternative health practitioners, and a past history of having sought information from sources on the internet or alternative health practitioners.[10]

Rather than being low-information parents, these are parents who are, if anything, less selective in choosing the sources they get information from. Rather than using information arrived at through the scientific method, they have also incorporated information from websites, alternative health practitioners, and religious leaders.

21 The Anti-vaccine Parent

Who is the typical "anti-vax" parent? What motivates them to disregard the advice of physicians, scientists, and public health officials? What do they value? Whom do they see as their peers? And how has their thinking gone astray? We have looked at cognitive effects, such as biased assimilation, the credibility heuristic, selective perception, the Dunning-Kruger effect, and backfire effects. We have also looked at how the availability of misinformation can lead people astray. We have examined at length the arguments made by major figures in the anti-vaccine movement, such as Andrew Wakefield, Robert F. Kennedy Jr., Robert Sears, and the Geiers. We have examined the demographics and religious beliefs of anti-vaccine activists and their historical predecessors. What does this all add up to? Let's paint a portrait of typical anti-vaccine parents, based on what we've learned them. This exercise isn't intended to set up straw men that will be easy for us to knock down, but rather to give us a concrete image of those to whom we can direct messaging.

Anti-vaccine parents are deeply concerned with being good parents. They are college educated and usually members of the middle class. They have read multiple parenting books and perhaps belong to parenting groups in their neighborhood or online. They have made decisions, in conjunction with discussions with their peers, about what kinds of parents to be. Breast or bottle feed? Public or private school? They may see themselves as "crunchy" parents, who are interested in "attachment" or "natural" parenting.

Let's give them names: Jim and Jenny, who live in Measlton, Michigan. One day Jenny sees a discussion in the Facebook group Measlton Moms. One parent says, "I went to the pediatrician and they wanted to vaccinate my baby. I said no. I don't want them injecting toxins into my baby." Another parent chimes in: "My daughter is vaccine injured. After she got the MMR shot, she had a fever for three days and then had seizures."

These stories alarm Jim and Jenny. They want to learn more before making a decision. Jim researches articles on websites like Natural News and InfoWars. Jenny finds books on Amazon. Some of what they read is alarming. Claims of medical fraud and cover-ups. Toxins that poison the blood being injected into children. Comparisons to Nazi doctors experimenting on children. Jim's cousin weighs in when she's visiting one day: "I didn't vaccinate my kids. Look how healthy they are." Rather than appealing to science, these sources appealed to moral concerns.

Moral foundations theory is a theory from social psychology meant to explain the variations in how people respond to moral arguments.[1] It posits that moral arguments tend to be based on certain foundations: concerns about care or harm, about fairness, about loyalty, about authority, and about purity. Some research indicates that these concerns respond best to arguments premised on *harm* or *fairness* and that conservatives tend also to respond to arguments based on authority, loyalty, and purity.

Jenny views herself as more liberal and is swayed by the arguments claiming that vaccines harm children and that it is unfair for the government to impose such a choice on her family. Jim, who views himself as more conservative, is swayed by these arguments, but also by the authoritative doctors and scientists that seems to support anti-vaccine views and by revulsion at the idea of compromising his child's purity by injecting it with foreign matter. They make what they feel is the right choice.

When Jenny takes the baby to its checkup with the pediatrician, Dr. Smith brings up its vaccine schedule. Jenny refuses and has come armed with information she's pulled from her sources on the internet and in books. She insists that there's mercury in vaccines that causes autism. She lists chemicals with long names that are in vaccines. Dr. Smith is taken aback. She agrees to delay but will try to persuade Jenny again at the next office visit.

At the next office visit, Dr. Smith has come prepared with responses to the anti-vaccine claims made by her patient. However, for every answer she can provide, Jenny has a rejoinder. The pediatrician is again delayed in vaccinating. Jenny feels ambushed by Dr. Smith. "I've done my research," she says. "As a mother, I know what's best for my own child, better than anyone else."

Jim and Jenny feel they've done their best for their child. They identified a potential danger, did research, and avoided that danger, which is the duty of good parents, after all. When Dr. Smith tried to convince them with facts and data alone, she failed because Jim and Jenny knew they shouldn't just trust whatever the pediatrician says. Long gone are the days of paternalism when the doctor knows best and a patient should simply listen and do what they're told. Jim and Jenny are active in their own health care and that of their children.

What could Dr. Smith have done to convince Jenny to go ahead with vaccination? What can municipalities, neighbors, and friends do to help Jim and Jenny make better choices?

Dr. Smith was operating from an information-deficit model. She believed that Jim and Jenny simply didn't have enough information. However, Jim and Jenny have more than enough information. It's just bad information. The bad information came from people whom Jim and Jenny trusted, friends and family. The good information came from an authority figure.

Imagine how this scenario would have played out if someone on the Measlton Moms Facebook group had stepped forward after that initial post to say "I had all three vaccinated, and they're doing great." Or if there had been another post with a picture of a smiling child with the caption "She just got her 24-month booster shots!" Perhaps if the sources that presented themselves when Jim and Jenny set out to do research had been better, they might have stopped themselves. Jim may have been directed to *New Scientist, Scientific American,* or another mostly reliable source, rather than to InfoWars and Natural News. Amazon's algorithm may have directed Jenny to books by Paul Offit, rather than to books by vaccine denialists.

Jim and Jenny's anti-vaccine stance arose in concert with many of the human tendencies, biases, and shortcuts of thinking that we've discussed before. People we know are more trustworthy than people we don't know. Statistics are less convincing than stories. Establishment authorities, such as physicians and federal agencies, engender distrust. Chemicals and substances with long and unpronounceable names can be frightening. We fear that putting things that are not natural into our bodies will make us impure. How we view ourselves and how we appear to our peers informs what we view as good parenting.

Now that Jim and Jenny have been convinced they've done the right thing, can their minds be changed? Has someone who was anti-vaccine ever changed their mind?

22   What Changes Minds about Vaccines?

In a blog post on the website Medium, Christine Vigeant, a scholar of philosophy and German studies, told the story of how she went from being against vaccines to changing her mind. She and her husband saw themselves as "crunchy" parents. They refused all childhood vaccinations. She sought advice from other parents who had adopted similar crunchy parenting techniques, and none of them vaccinated on schedule either. People critical of her decision seemed simply to be unwilling to challenge the status quo.

What changed Vigeant's mind was a friend on Facebook who was a part of many of the same parenting communities and who nonjudgmentally shared positive information about having her own children vaccinated. Gradually, by listening and asking questions, her friend was able to convince her that a lot of what she had believed about vaccines was wrong. Changing her mind took courage and open mindedness.[1]

Kristen O'Meara, a special-needs teacher, spoke to the *New York Post* about changing her mind about vaccines. She also saw her family as crunchy. They were better, in some ways, than the herds of people who never questioned the status quo or what medical officials told them. She sought out books and articles that confirmed her beliefs.

In 2015 her entire family came down with rotavirus, a vaccine-preventable illness. She became aware of the Disneyland measles outbreak. She had falsified a religious exemption for one of her daughters to enter a preschool but wondered if she should do it again. Then she decided that she would seek information that disconfirmed her beliefs. She read books by Seth Mnookin and Paul Offit and finally changed her mind.[2]

More stories about parents who went from being anti-vaccine to being pro-vaccine can be found on the website of the vaccine-advocacy group Voices for Vaccines. Chrissy, who was into healthy food and natural living, discovered anti-vaccine information on the internet. She stopped vaccinating her children after her first developed pertussis, despite being vaccinated against it. She felt justified, having done extensive reading on the internet. When she saw Jenny McCarthy on *Oprah* describing the symptoms of autism that matched some of the behaviors of her oldest child, she felt validated.

Eventually with a health scare during the birth of her second child, she decided to reevaluate her beliefs and seek out pro-vaccine information. She, too, read books by Seth Mnookin and Paul Offit, changed her mind, and had her children and herself vaccinated.[3]

Mary Miller, convinced that she was doing the best for her children, refused vaccination. She began to question her beliefs while working as a contractor at a hospital. She started to wonder how medicine worked and began to read books on vaccines. She had a health scare with chickenpox in one of her older children, and then when she became pregnant with a third child, she changed her mind and caught all her children up on their vaccine schedules.[4]

Megan Sandlin became involved in crunchy parenting and discovered that many of her crunchy friends did not vaccinate. She did internet research, reading vaccine inserts, and anti-vaccine websites. Her community cheered her on. She noticed that many of her anti-vaccine friends also posted about conspiracy theories that she didn't believe in, such as chemtrails. As a skeptic she continued doing reading and research on the internet, gradually finding her way to more reliable sources. For this, she lost many of her friends, who then blocked her on social media.[5]

Maranda Dynda followed the suggestion of a home-birth midwife to research vaccines. Dynda read websites critical of vaccination and became staunchly anti-vaccine. However, although she had become skeptical of medicine, she had always considered herself to be pro-science. She started to question the beliefs of some of her anti-vaccine friends, such as AIDS denialism, FEMA death camps, and essential oils. She continued her research, finding better resources, and changed her mind. She, too, lost friends.[6]

Ashley Chapman (a pseudonym) changed her mind when she watched her child come down with a serious case of croup that required hospitalization; she was terrified and embarrassed when she was asked whether her daughter was up to date on her immunizations.[7]

Courtney Allen saw herself as a "crunchy momma" and became deeply involved in reading and sharing information from anti-vaccine sources—until she saw a Facebook video made by a mother. The mother's child had contracted whooping cough, and as she filmed it struggling to breath, she pleaded that any viewer vaccinate their children. Allen's heart broke watching the pain of mother and child. Allen began doing more research, this time not just seeking out anti-vaccine information but reading pro-vaccine sources. She changed her mind.[8]

Ingvar Ingvarsson followed the advice he received from a health-food store not to vaccinate. That was until he became a nurse and started to work with older patients who had suffered from what are now vaccine-preventable diseases, such as measles and polio. These experiences led him to reevaluate his stance, and eventually he had his children vaccinated.[9]

These stories share some common themes. Parents build support networks with other parents with similar ideas about parenting. They seek information about vaccination and are directed to sources of information that seem to indicate that vaccines are unsafe. They feel they have done their research. Then something happens to change their views. They interact with a kind stranger who answers their questions. They connect with someone who was blinded by measles or paralyzed by polio. Their family suffers an illness, and they see how vulnerable they are. This leads them to do more research, seeking sources of information outside of those that confirm what they already believe.

We can take a few lessons from this. *People change their own minds; we can't do it for them.* We can hope to inspire our neighbors to do more and better research by being kind and supportive to and good role models for them. We can't hope to change their minds by making fun of them or forcing information down their throats. *Doing your own research isn't a bad thing, so long as you use good sources.* Each of these parents prided themselves on questioning the status quo and doing their own independent research. That research led them to anti-vaccine misinformation, but it also led them away from it. Being skeptical and questioning authority are admirable qualities. However, searching out information must be coupled with searching out *good* information. Helping people learn which sources are reliable will always be better than just presenting them with facts. *The anti-vaccine community will often drop support for those who leave it.* As good neighbors and friends, we should accept the burden of being a larger part of someone's social support network when that happens. Shunning has been an effective and painful tool of social control for centuries. *Building trust and acting with kindness are important tools in the fight for public health.* We don't all have medical degrees or posts in the government that allow us to speak from positions from authority, but we do have positions in the lives of others that allow us to speak to them as peers, neighbors, and members of the same communities.

Revisiting Jim and Jenny, we now know that the key to engaging them on vaccines is to treat them with respect and kindness. We can show them that we share many of the same values, that we attend the same mosque, that we have made many of the same parenting choices. We can show that our own children are healthy and relate that we have rewarded them for behaving well during a pediatrician visit to be vaccinated. We can answer Jim and Jenny's questions and patiently point them to sources they may not have considered.

Conclusions

Human life has always been stalked by disease. For bacteria, viruses, and parasites, our bodies and our cells are perfect incubators. Every life saved and every quantum of suffering avoided by a vaccine is the legacy of all the physicians and scientists who have ever devoted themselves to developing or disseminating these life-saving technologies. The anti-vaccination movement has worked its way into the public discourse, motivated by compassion and distrust of authority, experts, corporations, and governments.

So far, the degree of its success has been limited, and the degree of the success of researchers has been great. Researchers' legacy—those who went on to live long lives free from the diseases that plagued their ancestors—has become a part of a great human story about the power of ideas to conquer illness. That story is one that we must continue to tell. We should join voices with those researchers and in harmony sing praise to all of the life that is and was because of human invention and determination, and we should sing louder than those who sing out of key.

When public health workers soon eliminate polio and the suffering it inflicted becomes a memory we can learn about only in books and videos, it will become still harder to convince parents and patients of the importance of vaccination. The very presence of those who oppose vaccination are in that way a testament the effectiveness of vaccines. Just as the first anti-vaccine movements arose in the decades following the reduction of smallpox to a rare disease, the healthier we become, the harder we will need to work to preserve that health, as well as the advancements we've made.

The goal of convincing all parents to vaccinate, as well as to evaluate the risks and benefits of vaccination based on evidence, is one that will almost certainly never be achieved but is eminently worth pursuing. It is but one component of the overall fight against disease, but it is an important one, and one that almost anyone can participate in even without a lab or a medical license. But to be most effective, pro-vaccine activists must base their efforts on methods that are known to work.

Public health advocates are well advised to study the evidence; to use effective strategies when implementing programs aimed at encouraging vaccination; to avoid online confrontations and individual fights; and to focus on positive, socially aware messaging. Finally, we should focus on finding ways to reduce costs and increase access to vaccination for those who are currently undervaccinated but do not want to be.

The anti-vaccine movements of the nineteenth, twentieth, and twenty-first centuries have been motivated at their hearts by the desire to be a good parent and do what's best for one's children. This desire has been twisted by misinformation distributed by alternative health practitioners seeking to break up evidence's monopoly on health care, civil libertarians who fear government overreach, lawyers intent on raiding the coffers of government, pharmaceutical companies and clients, unscrupulous doctors willing to lie in order to sell sham treatments, and conspiracy theorists spinning vast and imaginary webs of deceit.

The victory of truth over lies and of information over disinformation is not a foregone conclusion. It is up to each of us to actively work to ensure that politicians who understand the value of science are elected, that clinicians have enough tools to convince patients of the best course of action for their own and their children's health, and that appealing lies never gain victory over hard-fought truths.

Acknowledgments

I wish to thank my brother Charles Berman for his help in editing, researching, and planning this book; my friends Harry Leeds, Leah Otto, and Nancy Gonzales for helping to review the manuscript; and my colleague Jesus Segovia for helping to review the immunology in this book.

Notes

Introduction

1. R. M. Wolfe and L. K. Sharp, "Anti-Vaccinationists Past and Present," *BMJ* 325 (2002): 430–432.

2. B. Taylor, E. Miller, C. P. Farrington, M. C. Petropoulos, I. Favot-Mayaud, J. Li, et al. "Autism and Measles, Mumps, and Rubella Vaccine: No Epidemiological Evidence for a Causal Association," *Lancet* 353 (1999): 2026–2029; L. Dales, S. J. Hammer, and N. J. Smith, "Time Trends in Autism and in MMR Immunization Coverage in California," *JAMA* 285 (2001): 1183–1185.

Chapter 1

1. H. A. Hill, L. D. Elam-Evans, D. Yankey, J. A. Singleton, and Y. Kang, "Vaccination Coverage among Children Aged 19–35 Months—United States, 2016," *Morbidity and Mortality Weekly Report* 66 (2017): 1171–1177.

2. R. Seither, K. Calhoun, E. J. Street, J. Mellerson, C. L. Knighton, A. Tippins, et al., "Vaccination Coverage for Selected Vaccines, Exemption Rates, and Provisional Enrollment among Children in Kindergarten— United States, 2016–17 School Year," *Morbidity and Mortality Weekly Report* 66 (2017): 1073–1080.

3. H. J. Larson, A. de Figueiredo, Z. Xiahong, W. S. Schulz, P. Verger, I. G. Johnston, et al., "The State of Vaccine Confidence 2016: Global

Insights through a 67-Country Survey," *EBioMedicine* 12 (2016): 295–301.

4. "Child Vaccination Rates," OECD data, https://data.oecd.org/health care/child-vaccination-rates.htm. (Accessed Nov. 1, 2019.)

5. G. Godin, M. Conner, and P. Sheeran, "Bridging the Intention-Behaviour Gap: The Role of Moral Norm," *British Journal of Social Psychology* 44 (2005): 497–512.

6. National Cancer Institute, "HPV and Cancer," www.cancer.gov/about -cancer/causes-prevention/risk/infectious-agents/hpv-fact-sheet. (Accessed Nov. 1, 2019.)

7. G. Haber, R. M. Malow, and G. D. Zimet, "The HPV Vaccine Mandate Controversy," *Journal of Pediatric Adolescent Gynecology* 20 (2007): 325–331; J. Colgrove, "The Ethics and Politics of Compulsory HPV Vaccination," *New England Journal of Medicine* 355 (2006): 2389–2391.

8. D. M. Kahan, "Social Science: A Risky Science Communication Environment for Vaccines," *Science* 342 (2013): 53–54.

9. D. M. Casciotti, K. C. Smith, L. Andon, J. Vernick, A. Tsui, and A. C. Klassen, "Print News Coverage of School-Based Human Papillomavirus Vaccine Mandates," *Journal of School Health* 84 (2014): 71–81.

10. A. Pollack and S. Saul, "Merck to Halt Lobbying for Vaccine for Girls," *New York Times*, February 21, 2007.

11. R. Shenoy, "Controversial Autism Researcher Tells Local Somalis Disease Is Solvable," Minnesota Public Radio News, 2010.

12. T. F. Leslie, P. L. Delamater, and Y. T. Yang, "It Could Have Been Much Worse: The Minnesota Measles Outbreak of 2017," *Vaccine* 36 (2018): 1808–1810.

13. L. H. Sun, "Measles Outbreak in Minnesota Surpasses Last Year's Total for the Entire Country," *Washington Post*, May 26, 2017, www .washingtonpost.com/national/health-science/imams-in-us-take-on-the -anti-vaccine-movement-during-ramadan/2017/05/26/8660edc6-41ad -11e7-8c25-44d09ff5a4a8_story.html.

Notes 219

14. L. H. Sun, "Despite Measles Outbreak, Anti-Vaccine Activists in Minnesota Refuse to Back Down," *Washington Post*, August 21, 2017, www.washingtonpost.com/national/health-science/despite-measles-outbreak-anti-vaccine-activists-in-minnesota-refuse-to-back-down/2017/08/21/886cca3e-820a-11e7-ab27-1a21a8e006ab_story.html.

15. Vaccination reduces the odds of contracting measles on exposure but does not eliminate all risk. Rong-Gong Lin II, "How California Got More Children Vaccinated after the Disneyland Measles Outbreak," *Los Angeles Times*, April 13, 2017, www.latimes.com/local/lanow/la-me-vaccination-explainer-20170413-story.html.

16. D. Goldschmidt, "More Than 800 Cases of Measles in US, with NY Outbreak Continuing to Lead," CNN, May 13, 2019, www.cnn.com/2019/05/13/health/measles-update-cdc-800-cases/index.html.

17. B. Y. Lee, "With Measles Crisis, Washington State Now Limits Vaccine Exemptions," *Forbes*, May 12, 2019. www.forbes.com/sites/brucelee/2019/05/12/with-measles-crisis-washington-state-now-limits-vaccine-exemptions/.

18. L. Wamsley, "Washington State Senate Passes Bill Removing Exemption for Measles Vaccine," NPR, April 18, 2019, www.npr.org/2019/04/18/714713364/washington-state-senate-passes-bill-removing-exemption-for-measles-vaccine.

19. D. Goldschmidt, "New York County Takes 'Extremely Unusual' Step to Ban Unvaccinated Minors from Public Places amid Measles Outbreak," CNN, March 26, 2019, www.cnn.com/2019/03/26/health/rockland-new-york-measles-unvaccinated-ban-bn/index.html.

20. R. Sanchez and S. Almasy, "Judge Stops NY County from Barring Unvaccinated Minors in Public Places as Measles Outbreak Continues," CNN, April 5, 2019, www.cnn.com/2019/04/05/health/rockland-new-york-measles-ban-ruling/index.html.

21. BBC News, "Cruise Ship Quarantined over Measles Case," BBC, May 2, 2019, www.bbc.com/news/world-latin-america-48130848.

22. E. Holt, "Ukraine at Risk of Polio Outbreak," *Lancet* 381 (2013): 2244.

23. "Measles, War, and Health-Care Reforms in Ukraine," *Lancet* 392 (2018): 711.

24. D. A. Broniatowski, A. M. Jamison, S. Qi, L. Al Kulaib, T. Chen, A. Benton, et al., "Weaponized Health Communication: Twitter Bots and Russian Trolls Amplify the Vaccine Debate," *American Journal of Public Health* 108 (2018): 1378–1384.

25. D. N. Durrheim, N. S. Crowcroft, and P. M. Strebel, "Measles—the Epidemiology of Elimination," *Vaccine* 32 (2014): 6880–6883.

26. P. J. Hotez, "Texas and Its Measles Epidemics," *PLoS Medicine* 13 (2016): e1002153.

27. T. Ackerman, "Vaccine Exemptions on the Rise among Texas Students," *Houston Chronicle*, August 15, 2016 [cited October 17, 2018], www.houstonchronicle.com/news/houston-texas/houston/article /Vaccine-exemptions-on-the-rise-among-Texas-9142343.php.

Chapter 3

1. Voltaire, *Philosophical Letters: Letters concerning the English Nation* (North Chelmsford, MA: Courier Corporation, 2012).

2. Diseases that can be caught by exposure to another person.

3. E. A. Wrigley, R. S. Davies, J. E. Oeppen, and R. S. Schofield, "Mortality," in *English Population History from Family Reconstitution, 1580–1837* (Cambridge: Cambridge University Press, 1997), 198–353.

4. C. Hallett, "The Attempt to Understand Puerperal Fever in the Eighteenth and Early Nineteenth Centuries: The Influence of Inflammation Theory," *Medical History* 49 (2005): 1–28.

5. The thick makeup sometimes seen in depictions of the era likely became fashionable as a way to hide smallpox scars.

6. M. A. Ruffer, M. Armand Ruffer, and A. R. Ferguson, "Note on an Eruption Resembling That of Variola in the Skin of a Mummy of the Twentieth Dynasty (1200–1100 B.C.)," *Journal of Pathology and*

Bacteriology 15 (1911): 1–3; D. R. Hopkins, *Princes and Peasants: Smallpox in History* (Chicago: University of Chicago Press, 1985).

7. F. Fenner, R. Wittek, and K. R. Dumbell, "Other Orthopoxviruses," in *The Orthopoxviruses* (San Diego, CA: Academic Press, 1989), 303–315.

8. J. Needham, *Science and Civilisation in China*, vol. 6: *Biology and Biological Technology*, "Part 1: Botany" (Cambridge: Cambridge University Press, 1986).

9. A. Boylston, "The Origins of Inoculation," *Journal of the Royal Society of Medicine* 105 (2012): 309–313.

10. E. Timonius and J. Woodward, "An Account, or History, of the Procuring the Small Pox by Incision, or Inoculation; As It Has for Some Time Been Practised at Constantinople," *Philosophical Transactions of the Royal Society of London* 29 (1714): 72–82.

11. J. Jurin and A. A. Rusnock, *The Correspondence of James Jurin (1684–1750): Physician and Secretary to the Royal Society* (Amsterdam: Rodopi, 1996).

12. S. Ross, "*Scientist*: The Story of a Word," in *Nineteenth-Century Attitudes: Men of Science* (Dordrecht: Kluwer Academic, 1991), 1–39.

13. G. Pearson, *An Inquiry concerning the History of the Cowpox, Principally with a View to Supersede and Extinguish the Smallpox* (London: Printed for J. Johnson, 1798).

Chapter 4

1. P. C. Plett, "[Peter Plett and Other Discoverers of Cowpox Vaccination before Edward Jenner]," *Sudhoffs Archive* 90 (2006): 219–232 (article in German).

2. P. C. Plett, "[Peter Plett and Other Discoverers of Cowpox Vaccination]."

3. J. F. Hammarsten, W. Tattersall, and J. E. Hammarsten, "Who Discovered Smallpox Vaccination? Edward Jenner or Benjamin Jesty?,"

Transactions of the American Clinical and Climatological Association 90 (1979): 44–55.

4. E. M. Crookshank, *History and Pathology of Vaccination*, vols. 1–2 (1889).

5. E. Jenner, *An Inquiry into the Causes and Effects of the Variolae Vaccinae: A Disease Discovered in Some of the Western Counties of England, Particularly Gloucestershire, and Known by the Name of the Cow Pox* (1801).

6. J. Baron, "Early History of Vaccination," in *The Life of Edward Jenner MD* (Cambridge: Cambridge University Press, 2014), 121–160.

7. The two outer layers of the skin, comprised of the dermis and epidermis.

8. S. Riedel, "Edward Jenner and the History of Smallpox and Vaccination," *Baylor University Medical Center Proceedings* 18 (2005): 21–25.

9. This is the opposite of how science is done.

10. T. Fulford and D. Lee, "The Jenneration of Disease: Vaccination, Romanticism, and Revolution," *Studies in Romanticism* 39 (2000): 139.

11. B. Moseley, *A Treatise on the "lues Bovilla" or Cow Pox, by Benjamin Moseley, …* 2nd ed. (1805).

12. Mother of the Minotaur.

13. "The Compulsory Vaccination Act," *Lancet* 62 (1853): 631.

14. The practice of variolation continued into modern times and was found to be continued in some areas up until close to the eradication of smallpox.

Chapter 5

1. "The Compulsory Vaccination Act," *Lancet* 62 (1853): 631.

2. Heroic medicine was a practice that emphasized the draining of bodily fluids, such as blood and sweat, as a means of balancing bodily "humors."

3. E. J. Gibbs, *Our Medical Liberties, or The Personal Rights of the Subject, as Infringed by Recent and Proposed Legislation: Compromising Observations on*

the Compulsory Vaccination Act, the Medical Registration and Reform Bills, and the Maine Law (1854).

4. D. Porter and R. Porter, "The Politics of Prevention: Anti-Vaccinationism and Public Health in Nineteenth-Century England," *Medical History* 32 (1988): 231–252.

5. Originally, statistics was used as a means of analyzing information about the state, and the term is derived from the Latin for "council of the state."

6. Great Britain, General Board of Health, S. J. Simon, *Papers Relating to the History and Practice of Vaccination: Presented to Both Houses of Parliament by Command of Her Majesty* (1857).

7. R. R. Frerichs, "London Epidemiological Society: Origin of Society," www.ph.ucla.edu/epi/snow/LESociety.html.

8. Miasma was a theory of disease proposing that disease was caused by exposure to bad air.

9. R. Murugan, "Movement towards Personalised Medicine in the ICU," *Lancet Respiratory Medicine* 3 (2015): 10–12.

10. Science, unlike medicine, does not have professional regulatory bodies. There is no specific test one takes to become a scientist, and one does not need a PhD or other degree to publish in scientific journals. For this reason, medical school is considered to be a professional school, but graduate school, where many young scientists train, is not. A PhD is meant to demonstrate mastery of and contribution to a scholarly field, not grant permission to practice in it.

11. "Thomas Percival (1740–1804) Codifier of Medical Ethics," *JAMA* 194 (1965): 1319.

12. Although the population growth of humanity has been nonlinear, there is reason to be optimistic. Over time the number of people living in extreme poverty overall has decreased, and the number of people living in hunger has decreased. In many developed nations, the birth rate has stabilized or dropped below replacement levels.

13. These beliefs are not features of utilitarianism but specific beliefs held by Bentham. Many modern utilitarians do not hold them.

14. U. Henriques, "How Cruel Was the Victorian Poor Law?" *Historical Journal* 11 (1968): 365.

15. J. R. Poynter and N. C. Edsall, "The Anti-Poor Law Movement, 1834–44," *American Historical Review* 77 (1972): 1125.

16. N. Durbach, *Bodily Matters: The Anti-Vaccination Movement in England, 1853–1907* (Durham, NC: Duke University Press, 2005).

17. Recommended for a thorough history of the era: N. Durbach, *Bodily Matters.*

18. J. D. Swales, "The Leicester Anti-Vaccination Movement," *Lancet* 340 (1992): 1019–1021.

19. S. Williamson, "Anti-Vaccination Leagues," *Archives of Disease in Childhood* 59 (1984): 1195–1196.

20. D. L. Ross, "Leicester and the Anti-Vaccination Movement, 1853–1889," *Transactions of the Leicester Archaeological Historical Society* 43 (1967): 35–44.

21. R. M. Wolfe and L. K. Sharp, "Anti-Vaccinationists Past and Present," *BMJ* 325 (2002): 430–432.

22. W. K. Mariner, G. J. Annas, and L. H. Glantz, "Jacobson v. Massachusetts: It's Not Your Great-Great-Grandfather's Public Health Law," *American Journal of Public Health* 95 (2005): 581–590.

23. P. Darmon, "[The Beginnings of Vaccine Diffusion in France (1800–1850)]," *Bulletin de L'Académie Nationale de Médecine* 185 (2001): 767–776.

Chapter 6

1. Microorganisms are living things that are too small to be seen by the eye unaided by a tool such as the optical microscope, which makes things appear larger to the human eye.

2. R. Cheyne, "The Late Mr. R. R. Cheyne and the Preservation of Vaccine Lymph," *Lancet* 151 (1898): 894.

3. J. J. Kinyoun, "The Action of Glycerin on Bacteria in the Presence of Cell Exudates," *Journal of Experimental Medicine* 7 (1905): 725–732.

4. D. A. Henderson, "The Eradication of Smallpox," *Scientific American* 235 (1976): 25–33.

5. L. H. Collier, "The Development of a Stable Smallpox Vaccine," *Journal of Hygiene* 53 (1955): 76–101.

6. D. Baxby, "The Origins of Vaccinia Virus," *Journal of Infectious Diseases* 136 (1977): 453–455.

7. Bacteria are a domain of life consisting of an estimated one trillion species, most of which have not yet been discovered. They are single-celled organisms, which are smaller than human cells and do not have a type of cell structure, called a nucleus, that human cells have.

8. L. Pasteur, Chamberland, Roux, "Summary Report of the Experiments Conducted at Pouilly-le-Fort, Near Melun, on the Anthrax Vaccination, 1881," *Yale Journal of Biology and Medicine* 75 (2002): 59–62.

9. M. de la Durantaye, *A Brief History of the Small Pox Epidemic in Montreal from 1871 to 1880 and the Late Outbrkae* [sic] *of 1885: Containing a Concise Account of the Inoculation of Ancient Time, the Discovery and Advantage of Vaccination, Mortality from Small Pox from 1871 to 1880, Together with a Summary of the Record of the Principal Events, with Statistics of Mortality of the Late Outbreak in 1885* (1885).

10. F. Fenner et al., *Smallpox and Its Eradication* (Geneva: World Health Organization, 1988).

Chapter 7

1. Mahatma Ghandi, *A Guide to Health*, trans. A. Rama Iyer (S. Ganesan, 1921).

2. Ghandi, *Guide to Health*.

3. "Reminiscences of Gandhi: At Sabarmati," www.gandhi-manibhavan.org/eduresources/chap8.htm.

4. The idea is this: the virus is well suited to infecting human cells and poorly suited to infecting macaque cells—although it can infect them. After being passed from one macaque to another over multiple passages the virus will evolve to be more suited to the new host and less suited to the old host. The new virus, which is less dangerous to humans, will still produce immunity in humans but with much less risk.

5. D. M. Horstmann, "The Poliomyelitis Story: A Scientific Hegira," *Yale Journal of Biology and Medicine* 58 (1985): 79–90.

6. Then the National Foundation for Infantile Paralysis.

7. J. E. Juskewitch, C. J. Tapia, and A. J. Windebank, "Lessons from the Salk Polio Vaccine: Methods for and Risks of Rapid Translation," *Clinical and Translational Science* 3 (2010): 182–185.

8. A. Day, "'An American Tragedy': The Cutter Incident and Its Implications for the Salk Polio Vaccine in New Zealand, 1955–1960," *Health History* 11 (2009): 42–61.

9. M. Kulenkampff, J. S. Schwartzman, and J. Wilson, "Neurological Complications of Pertussis Inoculation," *Archives of Disease in Childhood* 49 (1974): 46–49.

10. Rosemary Fox ARL, "Society Should Compensate for Brain Damage," *Birmingham Post* 10 (1973).

11. "Help for Victims of Immunizations," *BMJ* 1 (1973): 758–759.

12. G. Millward, "A Disability Act? The Vaccine Damage Payments Act 1979 and the British Government's Response to the Pertussis Vaccine Scare," *Social History of Medicine* 30 (2017): 429–447.

13. G. Amirthalingam, S. Gupta, and H. Campbell, "Pertussis Immunisation and Control in England and Wales, 1957 to 2012: A Historical Review," *Eurosurveillance* 18 (2013), www.ncbi.nlm.nih.gov/pubmed/24084340.

14. "TV Report on Vaccine Stirs Bitter Controversy," *Washington Post*, April 28, 1982, www.washingtonpost.com/archive/local/1982/04/28/tv

-report-on-vaccine-stirs-bitter-controversy/80d1fc8a-1012-4732-a517
-7976c86ab52d/.

15. V. Romanus, R. Jonsell, and S. O. Bergquist. "Pertussis in Sweden after the Cessation of General Immunization in 1979," *Pediatric Infectious Disease Journal* 6 (1987): 364–371.

16. P. E. Fine and J. A. Clarkson, "Individual versus Public Priorities in the Determination of Optimal Vaccination Policies," *American Journal of Epidemiology* 124 (1986): 1012–1020.

17. P. Huber, "Junk Science in the Courtroom," *Forbes*, July 8, 1991, www.overlawyered.com/articles/huber/junksci.html.

18. S. Engelberg, "Shortage of Whooping Cough Vaccine Is Seen," *New York Times*, December 14, 1984, www.nytimes.com/1984/12/14/us/shortage-of-whooping-cough-vaccine-is-seen.html.

19. G. L. Freed, S. L. Katz, and S. J. Clark, "Safety of Vaccinations: Miss America, the Media, and Public Health," *JAMA* 276 (1996): 1869–1872.

20. HRSA, "What You Need to Know about the National Vaccine Injury Compensation Program," September 2016, www.hrsa.gov/sites/default/files/vaccinecompensation/resources/84521booklet.pdf.

21. L. Cheng and W. Cheng, "Language Modeling for Legal Proof," in *Proceedings of 2010 IEEE International Conference on Intelligent Systems and Knowledge Engineering (ISKE)* (researchgate.net, 2010), 533–537.

22. United States Court of Appeals for the Federal Circuit, *Margaret Althen v. Secretary of Health and Human Services*, www.cafc.uscourts.gov/sites/default/files/opinions-orders/04-5146.pdf.

23. V. R. Walker, "Case Model: Werderitsh," LLT Lab, October 1, 2015, www.lltlab.org/case-model-werderitsh/.

24. P. A. Offit, "Vaccines and Autism Revisited—the Hannah Poling Case," *New England Journal of Medicine* 358 (2008): 2089–2091.

25. E. J. Woo, R. Ball, A. Bostrom, S. V. Shadomy, L. K. Ball, G. Evans, et al., "Vaccine Risk Perception among Reporters of Autism after

Vaccination: Vaccine Adverse Event Reporting System, 1990–2001," *American Journal of Public Health* 94 (2004): 990–995.

26. M. J. Goodman and J. Nordin, "Vaccine Adverse Event Reporting System Reporting Source: A Possible Source of Bias in Longitudinal Studies," *Pediatrics* 117 (2006): 387–390.

27. James R. Laidler, "Chelation and Autism," web.archive.org/web /20060423090641/www.neurodiversity.com/weblog/article/14/che lation-autism.

28. National Vaccine Program Office, Assistant Secretary for Health (ASH), "About the National Vaccine Program Office (NVPO)," www.hhs .gov/nvpo/about/index.html.

29. CDC, "Vaccine Information Statement: Inactivated Influenza Vaccine," www.cdc.gov/vaccines/hcp/vis/vis-statements/flu.pdf.

30. T. C. Davis, D. D. Fredrickson, C. L. Arnold, J. T. Cross, S. G. Humiston, K. W. Green, et al., "Childhood Vaccine Risk/Benefit Communication in Private Practice Office Settings: A National Survey," *Pediatrics* 107 (2001): E17.

Chapter 8

1. S. Hnilicova, K. Babinska, H. Celusakova, D. Filcikova, P. Kemenyova, and D. Ostatnikova, "Autism Etiology, Screening and Diagnosis," *Pathophysiology* 25 (2018): 193–194.

2. L. Kanner, "Autistic Disturbances of Affective Contact," *Nervous Child: Journal of Psychopathology, Psychotherapy, Mental Hygiene, and Guidance of the Child* 2 (1943): 217–250.

3. S. L. Smalley, R. F. Asarnow, and M. A. Spence, "Autism and Genetics: A Decade of Research," *Archives of General Psychiatry* 45 (1988): 953–961.

4. G. B. Schaefer and N. J. Mendelsohn, "Clinical Genetics Evaluation in Identifying the Etiology of Autism Spectrum Disorders," *Genetics in Medicine* 10 (2008): 301.

5. J. H. Miles, "Autism Spectrum Disorders—A Genetics Review," *Genetics in Medicine* 13 (2011): 278–294.

6. D. Bai, B. H. K Yip, G. C. Windham, A. Sourander, R. Francis, R. Yoffe, et al., "Association of Genetic and Environmental Factors with Autism in a 5-Country Cohort," *JAMA Psychiatry* (2019), doi:10.1001/jamapsychiatry.2019.1411.

7. Interestingly, the opposite is true in dogs. Almost all of the variation in the size of dogs comes down to a single gene.

8. S. De Rubeis, X. He, A. P. Goldberg, C. S. Poultney, K. Samocha, A. E. Cicek, et al. "Synaptic, Transcriptional, and Chromatin Genes Disrupted in Autism," *Nature* 515 (2014): 209–215.

9. W. Jones and A. Klin, "Attention to Eyes Is Present but in Decline in 2-6-Month-Old Infants Later Diagnosed with Autism," *Nature* 504 (2013): 427–431.

10. W. Jones, K. Carr, and A. Klin, "Absence of Preferential Looking to the Eyes of Approaching Adults Predicts Level of Social Disability in 2-Year-Old Toddlers with Autism Spectrum Disorder," *Archives of General Psychiatry* 65 (2008): 946–954.

11. R. Loomes, L. Hull, and W. P. L. Mandy, "What Is the Male-to-Female Ratio in Autism Spectrum Disorder? A Systematic Review and Meta-analysis," *Journal of the American Academy of Child Adolescent Psychiatry* 56 (2017): 466–474.

Chapter 9

1. Retraction is a fairly rare move and does not occur simply when a paper has been shown to be wrong, and it should not occur, for political reasons. According to the Committee on Publication Ethics, a retraction should only occur when editors have "clear evidence that the findings are unreliable, either as a result of misconduct, or honest error," that the findings have been previously published, that the paper constitutes plagiarism, or that the paper reports unethical research. Retraction is

intended as a means of correcting the literature when a grievous error occurs. Almost always the retracted paper remains available, but the reasons for retraction are specified. Discussion of the paper itself should be preceded with the knowledge that the scientific community and editors of the *Lancet* found the paper to meet these strict requirements for retraction. See COPE, "COPE's Retraction Guidelines," publicationethics.org /newsevents/cope%E2%80%99s-retraction-guidelines. (Accessed November 13, 2019.)

2. The Editors of the *Lancet*, "Retraction—Ileal-Lymphoid-Nodular Hyperplasia, Non-specific Colitis, and Pervasive Developmental Disorder in Children," *Lancet* 375 (2010): 445.

3. A. J. Wakefield, S. H. Murch, A. Anthony, J. Linnell, D. M. Casson, M. Malik, et al., "Ileal-Lymphoid-Nodular Hyperplasia, Non-specific Colitis, and Pervasive Developmental Disorder in Children," *Lancet* 351 (1998): 637–641.

4. N. Begg, M. Ramsay, J. White, and Z. Bozoky, "Media Dents Confidence in MMR Vaccine," *BMJ* 316 (1998): 561.

5. S. S. Coughlin, "Recall Bias in Epidemiologic Studies," *Journal of Clinical Epidemiology* 43 (1990): 87–91.

6. Robert T. Chen and Frank DeStefano, "Vaccine Adverse Events: Causal or Coincidental?" *Lancet* 51, no. 9103 (1998): 611–612.

7. M. A. Afzal, P. D. Minor, J. Begley, M. L. Bentley, E. Armitage, S. Ghosh, et al., "Absence of Measles-Virus Genome in Inflammatory Bowel Disease," *Lancet* 351 (1998): 646–647.

8. M. Kulenkampff, J. S. Schwartzman, and J. Wilson, "Neurological Complications of Pertussis Inoculation," *Archives of Disease in Childhood* 49 (1974): 46–49.

9. E. J. Gangarosa, A. M. Galazka, C. R. Wolfe, L. M. Phillips, R. E. Gangarosa, E. Miller, et al., "Impact of Anti-Vaccine Movements on Pertussis Control: The Untold Story," *Lancet* 351 (1998): 356–361.

10. J. Laurance, "I Was There When Wakefield Dropped His Bombshell," *Independent*, January 29, 2010, www.independent.co.uk/life-style

/health-and-families/health-news/i-was-there-when-wakefield-dropped
-his-bombshell-1882548.html.

11. Andrew Wakefield, quoted in B. Deer, "Focus—MMR: The Truth behind the Crisis," *Sunday Times*, February 22, 2004, briandeer.com /mmr/lancet-deer-2.htm.

12. D. Batty, "The Doctor Who Sparked the MMR Vaccination Debate," *Guardian*, March 27, 2008, www.theguardian.com/uk/2008/mar/27 /health.healthandwellbeing.

13. Institute of Medicine (US) Immunization Safety Review Committee, *Immunization Safety Review: Vaccines and Autism* (Washington, DC: National Academies Press, 2010).

14. B. Deer, "Focus—MMR: The Truth behind the Crisis."

15. H. Hodgson, "A Statement by the Royal Free and University College Medical School and the Royal Free Hampstead NHS Trust," *Lancet* (2004): 824.

16. S. H. Murch, A. Anthony, D. H. Casson, M. Malik, M. Berelowitz, A. P. Dhillon, et al., "Retraction of an Interpretation," *Lancet* 363 (2004): 750.

17. *Jab* is slang for "vaccination" in the UK.

18. B. Deer, "Secrets of the MMR Scare: How the Vaccine Crisis Was Meant to Make Money," *BMJ* 342 (2011): c5258.

19. P. A. Offit, *Autism's False Prophets: Bad Science, Risky Medicine, and the Search for a Cure* (New York: Columbia University Press, 2010).

20. J. W. Lee, B. Melgaard, C. J. Clements, M. Kane, E. K. Mulholland, and J. M. Olivé, "Autism, Inflammatory Bowel Disease, and MMR Vaccine," *Lancet* 351 (1998): 905; author's reply, 908–909.

21. A control in this case would be a group of children who had received the MMR vaccine but did not display symptoms of developmental regression.

22. In this context, "blinded" does not mean that the researchers ought to have had their eyes gouged out. It is a technique used in scientific

studies to reduce bias effects by, for example, making sure that researchers do not know whether they're examining endoscope images from children with developmental delays or controls.

23. A. Nicoll, D. Elliman, and E. Ross, "MMR Vaccination and Autism, 1998," *BMJ* 316 (1998): 715–716.

24. World Health Organization, Expanded Programme on Immunization (EPI), "Association between Measles Infection and the Occurrence of Chronic Inflammatory Bowel Disease," *Weekly Epidemiological Record* 73 (1998): 33–39.

25. J. Metcalf, "Is Measles Infection Associated with Crohn's Disease?," *BMJ* 316 (1998): 166.

26. Science cannot prove a hypothesis to be wrong; it can only fail to confirm it.

27. B. Taylor, E. Miller, C. P. Farrington, M. C. Petropoulos, I. Favot-Mayaud, J. Li, et al., "Autism and Measles, Mumps, and Rubella Vaccine: No Epidemiological Evidence for a Causal Association," *Lancet* 353 (1999): 2026–2029.

28. E. Fombonne and S. Chakrabarti, "No Evidence for a New Variant of Measles-Mumps-Rubella–Induced Autism," *Pediatrics* 108 (2001): E58.

29. J. A. Kaye, M. del Mar Melero-Montes, and H. Jick, "Mumps, Measles, and Rubella Vaccine and the Incidence of Autism Recorded by General Practitioners: A Time-Trend Analysis," *BMJ* 322 (2001): 460–463.

30. A. Mäkelä, J. P. Nuorti, and H. Peltola, "Neurologic Disorders after Measles-Mumps-Rubella Vaccination," *Pediatrics* 110 (2002): 957–963.

31. B. Taylor, E. Miller, R. Lingam, N. Andrews, A. Simmons, and J. Stowe, "Measles, Mumps, and Rubella Vaccination and Bowel Problems or Developmental Regression in Children with Autism: Population Study," *BMJ* 324 (2002): 393–396.

32. M. Szumilas, "Explaining Odds Ratios," *Journal of the Canadian Academy of Child and Adolescent Psychiatry* 19 (2010): 227–229.

33. F. DeStefano, C. S. Price, and E. S. Weintraub, "Increasing Exposure to Antibody-Stimulating Proteins and Polysaccharides in Vaccines Is Not Associated with Risk of Autism," *Journal of Pediatrics* 163 (2013): 561–567.

34. L. E. Taylor, A. L. Swerdfeger, and G. D. Eslick, "Vaccines Are Not Associated with Autism: An Evidence-Based Meta-analysis of Case-Control and Cohort Studies," *Vaccine* 32 (2014): 3623–3629.

35. J. Lewis and T. Speers, "Misleading Media Reporting? The MMR Story," *Nature Reviews Immunology* 3 (2003): 913–918.

36. B. Dixon, "Triple Vaccine Fears Mask Media Efforts at Balance," *Current Biology* 12 (2002): R151–152.

37. Featuring a plaque with a flying pig on it.

38. J. Carrey, "The Judgment on Vaccines Is In???" *Huffington Post*, November 5, 2009, www.huffingtonpost.com/entry/the-judgment-on-vaccines_us_5b9c4fb4e4b03a1dcc7db886.

39. L. West, "Alicia Silverstone's Nutty New Parenting Book Is Anti-Vax, Anti-Diaper," *Jezebel*, April 23, 2014, https://jezebel.com/alicia-silverstones-nutty-new-parenting-book-is-anti-va-1566382435.

40. A. Merlan, "Here's a Fairly Comprehensive List of Anti-Vaccination Celebrities," *Jezebel*, June 30, 2015, https://jezebel.com/heres-a-fairly-comprehensive-list-of-anti-vaccination-c-1714760128.

41. E. Wyatt, "ABC Drama Takes on Science and Parents," *New York Times*, January 23, 2008, www.nytimes.com/2008/01/23/arts/television/23ston.html.

42. E. Wyatt, "ABC Show Will Go On, over Protest by Doctors," *New York Times*, January 29, 2008, www.nytimes.com/2008/01/29/business/media/29abc.html.

43. B. Fjæstad, "Why Journalists Report Science as They Do," in *Journalism, Science, and Society*, ed. Martin W. Bauer and Massimiano Bucchi (Abingdon: Routledge, 2007).

44. R. Rosenthal, "The File Drawer Problem and Tolerance for Null Results," *Psychological Bulletin* 86 (1979): 638–641.

45. S. O'Neill, H. T. P. Williams, T. Kurz, B. Wiersma, and M. Boykoff, "Dominant Frames in Legacy and Social Media Coverage of the IPCC Fifth Assessment Report," *Nature Climate Change* 5 (2015): 380.

46. M. Siegrist and G. Cvetkovich, "Better Negative Than Positive? Evidence of a Bias for Negative Information about Possible Health Dangers," *Risk Analysis* 21 (2001): 199–206.

47. A. Tversky and D. Kahneman, "Judgment under Uncertainty: Heuristics and Biases," *Science* 185 (1974): 1124–1131.

48. "Science Journalism Can Be Evidence-Based, Compelling—and Wrong," *Nature* 543 (2017): 150.

49. B. Deer, "How the Case against the MMR Vaccine Was Fixed," *BMJ* 342 (2011): c5347.

50. S. Boseley, "Andrew Wakefield Struck Off Register by General Medical Council," *Guardian*, May 24, 2010, www.theguardian.com/society /2010/may/24/andrew-wakefield-struck-off-gmc.

51. B. Deer, "Secrets of the MMR Scare: How the Vaccine Crisis Was Meant to Make Money," *BMJ* 342 (2011): c5258.

52. "Editorial: Wakefield's Article Linking MMR Vaccine and Autism Was Fraudulent," *BMJ* 342 (2011): c7452.

53. M. A. Roser, "British Doctor Resigns as Head of Austin Autism Center," *Austin American-Statesman*, September 1, 2012, www.statesman .com/article/20120901/NEWS/308998920.

54. A. Hannaford, M. Barajas, and S. Novack, "Autism Inc.: The Discredited Science, Shady Treatments, and Rising Profits behind Alternative Autism Treatments," *Texas Observer*, January 30, 2013, www .texasobserver.org/autism-inc-the-discredited-science-shady-treatments -and-rising-profits-behind-alternative-autism-treatments/.

55. M. Carey, "Is Andrew Wakefield's Strategic Autism Initiative Failing?," *Left Brain Right Brain*, March 3, 2015, https://leftbrainrightbrain .co.uk/category/orgs/strategic-autism-initiative/.

56. R. Shenoy, "Controversial Autism Researcher Tells Local Somalis Disease Is Solvable," Minnesota Public Radio News, 2010.

57. A. Hannaford, "Andrew Wakefield: Autism Inc.," *Guardian*, April 6, 2013, www.theguardian.com/society/2013/apr/06/what-happened-man -mmr-panic.

58. M. Ryzik, "Anti-Vaccine Film, Pulled from Tribeca Film Festival, Draws Crowd at Showing," *New York Times*, April 2, 2016, www.nytimes .com/2016/04/02/nyregion/anti-vaccine-film-pulled-from-tribeca-film -festival-draws-crowd-at-showing.html.

Chapter 10

1. P. Diethelm and M. McKee, "Denialism: What Is It and How Should Scientists Respond?" *European Journal of Public Health* 19 (2009): 2–4.

2. F. DeStefano, T. K. Bhasin, W. W. Thompson, M. Yeargin-Allsopp, and C. Boyle, "Age at First Measles-Mumps-Rubella Vaccination in Children with Autism and School-Matched Control Subjects: A Population-Based Study in Metropolitan Atlanta," *Pediatrics* 113 (2004): 259–266.

3. B. S. Hooker, "Measles-Mumps-Rubella Vaccination Timing and Autism among Young African American Boys: A Reanalysis of CDC Data," *Translational Neurodegeneration* 3 (2014): 16.

4. "Retraction: Measles-Mumps-Rubella Vaccination Timing and Autism among Young African American Boys: A Reanalysis of CDC Data," *Translational Neurodegeneration* 3 (2014): 22.

5. Minitab Blog Editor, "Analysis and Reanalysis: The Controversy behind MMR Vaccinations and Autism, Part 1," http://blog.minitab .com/blog/adventures-in-statistics-2/analysis-and-reanalysis3a-the -controversy-behind-mmr-vaccinations-and-autism2c-part-1.

6. Minitab Blog Editor, "Analysis and Reanalysis: The Controversy behind MMR Vaccinations and Autism, Part 2," http://blog.minitab .com/blog/adventures-in-statistics-2/analysis-and-reanalysis3a-the -controversy-behind-mmr-vaccinations-and-autism2c-part-2.

7. D. Gorsky, "Vaccine Whistleblower: An Antivaccine 'Exposé' Full of Sound and Fury, Signifying Nothing," *Science-Based Medicine*, August 24, 2015, https://sciencebasedmedicine.org/vaccine-whistleblower-an-antivaccine-expose-full-of-sound-and-fury-signifying-nothing/; Kevin Barry, *Vaccine Whistleblower: Exposing Autism Research Fraud at the CDC* (New York: Simon and Schuster, 2015).

8. To the degree that two people can be said to be friends when one is secretly recording the other.

9. E. Willingham, "A Congressman, a CDC Whistleblower, and an Autism Tempest in a Trashcan," *Forbes*, August 6, 2015, www.forbes.com /sites/emilywillingham/2015/08/06/a-congressman-a-cdc-whisteblower -and-an-autism-tempest-in-a-trashcan/.

10. M. Carey, "A Look at the Analysis Plan for DeStefano's MMR Study: No Evidence of Fraud," *Left Brain Right Brain*, October 16, 2014, https:// leftbrainrightbrain.co.uk/2014/10/16/a-look-at-the-analysis-plan-for -destefanos-mmr-study-no-evidence-of-fraud/.

11. The phenomenon of Nobel Prize winners endorsing various crank ideas is so common that it has received a name: "Nobel Disease." Over the years, Nobel Prize winners have supported or endorsed psychic mediums, Nazi racial theories, beliefs in ESP and paranormal phenomena, evolution denial, vitamin C megadosing, "quantum consciousness," cold fusion, global warming denial, alien abduction, a holographic talking raccoon, AIDS denial, and homeopathy. All of this goes to show that brilliance in one area does not mean credibility in *all* areas.

12. United States Court of Federal Claims, *Brian Hooker and Marcie Hooker, Parents of SRH, a Minor, v. Secretary of Health and Human Services, Respondent*, https://lbrbblog.files.wordpress.com/2016/07/hooker-vaccine-court.pdf.

13. MMR as given to the children in the 1998 *Lancet* paper did not contain thimerosal.

14. M. Carey, "Double Checking Brian Hooker's Story in VAXXED," *Left Brain Right Brain*, July 7, 2016, https://leftbrainrightbrain.co.uk/2016/07 /07/double-checking-brian-hookers-story-in-vaxxed/.

15. CDC, "Autism and Developmental Disabilities Monitoring (ADDM) Network," www.cdc.gov/ncbddd/autism/addm.html.

16. Orac, "The Antivaccine Movement Resurrects the Zombie That Is the 'Autism Epidemic,'" *Respectful Insolence*, March 31, 2014, https://respectfulinsolence.com/2014/03/31/the-antivaccine-movement-resurrects-the-zombie-2014/.

17. Ari LeVaux, "Meet the Controversial MIT Scientist Who Claims She Discovered a Cause of Gluten Intolerance," *Alternet*, February 27, 2014, www.alternet.org/food/meet-controversial-mit-scientist-who-claims-have-discovered-cause-gluten-sensitivty.

18. Such journals are a large problem in the life sciences. They prey on the publish-or-perish culture of science, wherein the quality of a publication is often less important than is the mere fact of its existence. Essentially, for a price, many of them will publish anything. I personally receive two to three emails a day asking me to publish in such and such new open-access journal. Open access itself is good because it allows greater unrestricted dissemination of research findings, but care must be taken to distinguish reputable from nonreputable journals.

19. R. Mesnage and M. N. Antoniou, "Facts and Fallacies in the Debate on Glyphosate Toxicity," *Frontiers in Public Health* 5 (2017): 316.

20. In a life-saving cancer surgery, carried out by highly trained physicians.

Chapter 11

1. P. A. Offit and C. A. Moser, "The Problem with Dr Bob's Alternative Vaccine Schedule," *Pediatrics* 123 (2009): e164–e169.

2. A. T. Glenny and H. J. Südmersen, "Notes on the Production of Immunity to Diphtheria Toxin," *Journal of Hygiene* 20 (1921): 176–220.

3. T. R. Ghimire, "The Mechanisms of Action of Vaccines Containing Aluminum Adjuvants: An In Vitro vs. In Vivo Paradigm," *Springerplus* 4 (2015): 181.

4. A. T. Glenny, G. A. H. Buttle, and M. F. Stevens, "Rate of Disappearance of Diphtheria Toxoid Injected into Rabbits and Guinea-Pigs: Toxoid Precipitated with Alum," *Journal of Pathology* 34 (1931): 267–275.

5. R. G. White, A. H. Coons, and J. M. Connolly, "Studies on Antibody Production. III. The Alum Granuloma," *Journal of Experimental Medicine* 102 (1955): 73–82.

6. N. W. Baylor, W. Egan, and P. Richman, "Aluminum Salts in Vaccines—US Perspective," *Vaccine* 20 (2002): S18–S23.

7. J. G. Dórea and R. C. Marques, "Infants' Exposure to Aluminum from Vaccines and Breast Milk during the First 6 Months," *Journal of Exposure Science and Environmental Epidemiology* 20 (2010): 598–601.

8. N. Chuchu, B. Patel, B. Sebastian, and C. Exley, "The Aluminium Content of Infant Formulas Remains Too High," *BMC Pediatrics* 13 (2013): 162.

9. R. E. Litov, V. S. Sickles, G. M. Chan, M. A. Springer, and A. Cordano, "Plasma Aluminum Measurements in Term Infants Fed Human Milk or a Soy-Based Infant Formula," *Pediatrics* 84 (1989): 1105–1107.

10. B. Flannery, S. B. Reynolds, L. Blanton, T. A. Santibanez, A. O'Halloran, P.-J. Lu, et al., "Influenza Vaccine Effectiveness against Pediatric Deaths, 2010–2014," *Pediatrics* 139 (2017): e20164244.

11. D. G. McNeil Jr., "Over 80,000 Americans Died of Flu Last Winter, Highest Toll in Years," *New York Times*, October 1, 2018, www.nytimes.com/2018/10/01/health/flu-deaths-vaccine.html.

12. K. A. Poehling, K. M. Edwards, G. A. Weinberg, P. Szilagyi, M. A. Staat, M. K. Iwane, et al. "The Underrecognized Burden of Influenza in Young Children," *New England Journal of Medicine* 355 (2006): 31–40.

13. NIH, National Institute of Neurological Disorders and Stroke, "Guillain-Barré Syndrome Fact Sheet," www.ninds.nih.gov/Disorders/Patient-Caregiver-Education/Fact-Sheets/Guillain-Barre-Syndrome-Fact-Sheet.

14. P. Haber, F. DeStefano, F. J. Angulo, J. Iskander, S. V. Shadomy, E. Weintraub, et al., "Guillain-Barré Syndrome following Influenza Vaccination," *JAMA* 292 (2004): 2478–2481.

15. W. K. Yih, E. Weintraub, and M. Kulldorff, "No Risk of Guillain-Barré Syndrome Found after Meningococcal Conjugate Vaccination in Two Large Cohort Studies," *Pharmacoepidemiology and Drug Safety*, December 6, 2012, 1359–1360.

16. S. B. Black, H. R. Shinefield, R. A. Hiatt, and B. H. Fireman, "Efficacy of Haemophilus Influenzae Type B Capsular Polysaccharide Vaccine," *Pediatric Infectious Disease Journal* 7 (1988): 149–156.

17. L. H. Harrison, C. V. Broome, A. W. Hightower, C. C. Hoppe, S. Makintubee, S. L. Sitze, et al., "A Day Care–Based Study of the Efficacy of Haemophilus B Polysaccharide Vaccine," *JAMA* 260 (1988): 1413–1418.

18. M. T. Osterholm, J. H. Rambeck, K. E. White, J. L. Jacobs, L. M. Pierson, J. D. Neaton, et al., "Lack of Efficacy of Haemophilus B Polysaccharide Vaccine in Minnesota," *JAMA* 260 (1988): 1423–1428.

19. E. D. Shapiro, T. V. Murphy, E. R. Wald, and C. A. Brady, "The Protective Efficacy of Haemophilus B Polysaccharide Vaccine," *JAMA* 260 (1988): 1419–1422.

20. D. J. Granoff, P. G. Shackelford, B. K. Suarez, M. H. Nahm, K. L. Cates, T. V. Murphy, et al., "Hemophilus Influenzae Type B Disease in Children Vaccinated with Type B Polysaccharide Vaccine," *New England Journal of Medicine* 315 (1986): 1584–1590.

21. R. S. Daum, S. K. Sood, M. T. Osterholm, J. C. Pramberg, P. D. Granoff, K. E. White, et al., "Decline in Serum Antibody to the Capsule of Haemophilus Influenzae Type B in the Immediate Postimmunization Period," *Journal of Pediatrics* 114 (1989): 742–747.

22. C. D. Marchant, E. Band, J. E. Froeschle, and P. H. McVerry, "Depression of Anticapsular Antibody after Immunization with Haemophilus Influenzae Type B Polysaccharide-Diphtheria Conjugate Vaccine," *Pediatric Infectious Disease Journal* 8 (1989): 508–511.

23. Institute of Medicine (US) Vaccine Safety Committee, K. R. Stratton, C. J. Howe, and R. B. Johnston Jr., *Haemophilus Influenzae Type B Vaccines* (Washington, DC: National Academies Press, 1994).

24. C.-Y. Fang, C.-C. Wu, C.-L. Fang, W.-Y. Chen, C.-L. Chen, "Long-Term Growth Comparison Studies of FBS and FBS Alternatives in Six Head and Neck Cell Lines," *PLoS One* 12 (2017): e0178960.

25. J. Dumont, D. Euwart, B. Mei, S. Estes, and R. Kshirsagar, "Human Cell Lines for Biopharmaceutical Manufacturing: History, Status, and Future Perspectives," *Critical Reviews in Biotechnology* 36 (2016): 1110–1122.

26. Mad cow disease is also known as bovine spongiform encephalopathy.

27. A. H. Peden, M. W. Head, D. L. Ritchie, J. E. Bell, and J. W. Ironside, "Preclinical vCJD after Blood Transfusion in a PRNP Codon 129 Heterozygous Patient," *Lancet* 364 (2004): 527–529.

28. B. S. Appleby, M. Lu, A. Bizzi, M. D. Phillips, S. M. Berri, M. D. Harbison, et al., "Iatrogenic Creutzfeldt-Jakob Disease from Commercial Cadaveric Human Growth Hormone," *Emerging Infectious Diseases* 19 (2013): 682–684.

29. About 270 pounds for those still stuck on non-SI units.

30. CDC, "Variant Creutzfeldt-Jakob Disease: vCJD Cases Reported in the US," page last reviewed October 9, 2018, www.cdc.gov/prions/vcjd /vcjd-reported.html.

31. CDC, "Immunization Schedules: Table 1: Recommended Child and Adolescent Immunization Schedule for Ages 18 Years or Younger, United States, 2019," page last reviewed February 5, 2019, www.cdc.gov /vaccines/schedules/hcp/imz/child-adolescent.html.

32. CDC, "Vaccines for Your Children: Who Sets the Immunization Schedule," page last reviewed March 8, 2012, www.cdc.gov/vaccines /parents/vaccine-decision/sets-schedule.html.

Chapter 12

1. K. Lauerman, "Correcting Our Record," Salon.com, January 16, 2011, www.salon.com/2011/01/16/dangerous_immunity/.

2. Again, science is almost always conducted assuming that the null hypothesis, that there is no effect, is true.

3. Orac, "Salon.com Flushes Its Credibility Down the Toilet," *Respectful Insolence* (blog), June 17, 2005, http://oracknows.blogspot.com/2005/06 /saloncom-flushes-its-credibility-down.html.

4. "Robert F. Kennedy Junior's Completely Dishonest Thimerosal Article," *Skeptico* (blog), June 20, 2005, https://skeptico.blogs.com/skeptico /2005/06/robert_f_kenned.html.

5. "Lies, Damned Lies, and Quote Mining," *Skeptico* (blog), June 29, 2005, https://skeptico.blogs.com/skeptico/2005/06/lies_damn_lies_.html.

6. Robert F. Kennedy Jr., "The True History behind Salon's Retraction of My 'Deadly Immunity' Article," Children's Health Defense, May 1, 2015, https://worldmercuryproject.org/news/salons-retraction-deadly-immunity -article-real-reason-behind/.

7. Mercury is naturally occurring, and like all elements higher in the periodic table than iron, is formed only in supernovae.

8. World Health Organization, International Programme on Chemical Safety, "Methylmercury / published under the joint sponsorship of the United Nations Environment Programme, the International Labour Organisation, and the World Health Organization" (1990), www.who .int/iris/handle/10665/38082.

9. The unit used for measuring blood pressure in a physiological context is still mmHg, or millimeters of mercury, which are roughly equal to 0.134 kPa in SI units. Early manometers, or pressure meters, used the height in mm of a mercury column to measure pressure. The two numbers (ex 120/80) represent the points at which while pressure is released from occluding the brachial artery, sounds become audible due to turbulent flow as the BP is able to overcome the cuff pressure to open the artery, and the point at which pressure during diastole is adequate to overcome the cuff pressure.

10. R. A. Bernhoft, "Mercury Toxicity and Treatment: A Review of the Literature," *Journal of Environmental and Public Health* (2012): 460508.

11. L. K. Ball, R. Ball, and R. D. Pratt, "An Assessment of Thimerosal Use in Childhood Vaccines," *Pediatrics* 107 (2001): 1147–1154.

12. G. L. Freed, M. C. Andreae, A. E. Cowan, and S. L. Katz, "The Process of Public Policy Formulation: The Case of Thimerosal in Vaccines," *Pediatrics* 109 (2002): 1153–1159.

13. T. W. Clarkson, L. Magos, and G. J. Myers, "The Toxicology of Mercury—Current Exposures and Clinical Manifestations," *New England Journal of Medicine* 349 (2003): 1731–1737.

14. M. E. Pichichero, E. Cernichiari, J. Lopreiato, and J. Treanor. "Mercury Concentrations and Metabolism in Infants Receiving Vaccines Containing Thiomersal: A Descriptive Study," *Lancet* 360 (2002): 1737–1741.

15. G. L. Freed, M. C. Andreae, A. E. Cowan, and S. L. Katz, "The Process of Public Policy Formulation: The Case of Thimerosal in Vaccines," *Pediatrics* 109 (2002): 1153–1159.

16. CDC, Vaccine Safety, "Timeline: Thimerosal in Vaccines (1999–2010)," March 21, 2017, www.cdc.gov/vaccinesafety/concerns/thimerosal/timeline.html.

17. L. K. Ball, R. Ball, and R. D. Pratt, "An Assessment of Thimerosal Use in Childhood Vaccines," *Pediatrics* 107 (2001): 1147–1154.

18. T. Verstraeten, R. L. Davis, F. DeStefano, T. A. Lieu, P. H. Rhodes, S. B. Black, et al., "Safety of Thimerosal-Containing Vaccines: A Two-Phased Study of Computerized Health Maintenance Organization Databases," *Pediatrics* 112 (2003): 1039–1048.

19. P. Stehr-Green, P. Tull, M. Stellfeld, P.-B. Mortenson, and D. Simpson, "Autism and Thimerosal-Containing Vaccines: Lack of Consistent Evidence for an Association," *American Journal of Preventive Medicine* 25 (2003): 101–106.

20. Institute of Medicine (US) Immunization Safety Review Committee, *Immunization Safety Review: Vaccines and Autism* (Washington, DC: National Academies Press, 2010).

21. W. W. Thompson, C. Price, B. Goodson, D. K. Shay, P. Benson, V. L. Hinrichsen, et al., "Early Thimerosal Exposure and Neuropsychological Outcomes at 7 to 10 Years," *New England Journal of Medicine* 357 (2007): 1281–1292; C. S. Price, W. W. Thompson, B. Goodson, E. S. Weintraub, L. A. Croen, V. L. Hinrichsen, et al., "Prenatal and Infant Exposure to Thimerosal from Vaccines and Immunoglobulins and Risk of Autism," *Pediatrics* 126 (2010): 656–664; A. E. Tozzi, P. Bisiacchi, V. Tarantino, B. De Mei, L. D'Elia, F. Chiarotti, et al., "Neuropsychological Performance 10 Years after Immunization in Infancy with Thimerosal-Containing Vaccines," *Pediatrics* 123 (2009): 475–482.

22. A. Phillip, L. H. Sun, and L. Bernstein, "Vaccine Skeptic Robert Kennedy Jr. Says Trump Asked Him to Lead Commission on 'Vaccine Safety,'" *Washington Post*, January 10, 2017, www.washingtonpost.com/politics /trump-to-meet-with-proponent-of-debunked-tie-between-vaccines-and -autism/2017/01/10/4a5d03c0-d752-11e6-9f9f-5cdb4b7f8dd7_story .html.

23. Karie Youngdahl, "President-Elect Donald Trump and Vaccines," History of Vaccines, November 10, 2016, www.historyofvaccines.org /trump-and-vaccines.

24. M. Vazquez, "Trump Now Says Parents Must Vaccinate Children in Face of Measles Outbreak," CNN, April 26, 2019, www.cnn.com/2019 /04/26/politics/donald-trump-measles-vaccines/index.html.

25. C. A. Foster, "The $100,000 Vaccine Challenge: Another Method of Promoting Anti-Vaccination Pseudoscience," *Vaccine* 35 (2017): 3905–3906.

Chapter 13

1. For more information, see the rest of the book you're reading right now.

2. T. Ghianni, "Swapping Chicken Pox–Infected Lollipops Illegal," Reuters, November 12, 2011, www.reuters.com/article/us-chickenpox -lollipops-idUSTRE7AB0SW20111112.

3. E. E. Stevens, T. E. Patrick, and R. Pickler, "A History of Infant Feeding," *Journal of Perinatal Education* 18 (2009): 32–39.

4. P. Van de Perre, "Transfer of Antibody via Mother's Milk," *Vaccine* 21 (2003): 3374–3376.

5. W. B. Jonas, T. J. Kaptchuk, and K. Linde, "A Critical Overview of Homeopathy," *Annals of Internal Medicine* 138 (2003): 393–399.

6. R. T. Mathie, J. Frye, and P. Fisher, "Homeopathic Oscillococcinum® for Preventing and Treating Influenza and Influenza-like Illness," *Cochrane Database of Systematic Reviews* 1 (2015): CD001957.

7. Carmen, "Natural Vaccination Alternatives for You and Your Kids," Off the Grid News, September 24, 2012, www.offthegridnews.com/alternative-health/natural-vaccination-alternatives-for-you-and-your-kids/.

8. L. Pauling, *Vitamin C, the Common Cold, and the Flu* (San Francisco: W. H. Freeman, 1970); E. Cameron and L. C. Pauling, *Cancer and Vitamin C: A Discussion of the Nature, Causes, Prevention, and Treatment of Cancer with Special Reference to the Value of Vitamin C* (Linus Pauling Institute of Science and Medicine, 1979); L. Pauling, "Vitamin C and the Common Cold," *Canadian Medical Association Journal* 105 (1971): 448.

9. L. Pauling, "Orthomolecular Psychiatry: Varying the Concentrations of Substances Normally Present in the Human Body May Control Mental Disease," *Science* 160 (1968): 265–271.

10. "Megavitamin and Orthomolecular Therapy in Psychiatry: Excerpts from a Report of the American Psychiatric Association Task Force on Vitamin Therapy in Psychiatry," *Nutrition Reviews* 32 (1974): 44–47; Nutrition Committee, Canadian Paediatric Society, "Megavitamin and Megamineral Therapy in Childhood," *Canadian Medical Association Journal* 143 (1990): 1009–1013.

11. "How to Detoxify from a Vaccine," Season Johnson, March 20, 2018, www.seasonjohnson.com/how-to-detoxify-from-a-vaccine/.

12. J. A. Astin, "Why Patients Use Alternative Medicine: Results of a National Study," *JAMA* 279 (1998): 1548–1553.

13. M. Siahpush, "Why Do People Favour Alternative Medicine?" *Australian and New Zealand Journal of Public Health* 23 (1999): 266–271.

14. F. L. Bishop, L. Yardley, and G. T. Lewith, "Why Consumers Maintain Complementary and Alternative Medicine Use: A Qualitative Study," *Journal of Alternative and Complementary Medicine* 16 (2010): 175–182.

15. F. L. Bishop, L. Yardley, and G. T. Lewith, "Why Do People Use Different Forms of Complementary Medicine? Multivariate Associations between Treatment and Illness Beliefs and Complementary Medicine Use," *Psychology and Health* 21 (2006): 683–698.

16. M. O'Keefe and S. Coat, "Increasing Health-Care Options: The Perspectives of Parents Who Use Complementary and Alternative Medicines," *Journal of Paediatrics and Child Health* 46 (2010): 296–300.

17. R. Jütte, "The Early History of the Placebo," *Complementary Therapies in Medicine* 21 (2013): 94–97.

18. A. Branthwaite and P. Cooper, "Analgesic Effects of Branding in Treatment of Headaches," *BMJ* 282 (1981): 1576–1578.

19. D. E. Moerman and W. B. Jonas, "Deconstructing the Placebo Effect and Finding the Meaning Response," *Annals of Internal Medicine* 136 (2002): 471–476.

20. M. Adams, W. J. Blumenfeld, R. Castaneda, H. W. Hackman, M. L. Peters, and X. Zuniga, *Readings for Diversity and Social Justice* (Psychology Press, 2000).

21. D. A. Wolfe and E. J. Mash, eds., *Behavioral and Emotional Disorders in Adolescents: Nature, Assessment, and Treatment* (New York: Guilford Press, 2008).

22. A. Badaru, D. M. Wilson, L. K. Bachrach, P. Fechner, L. M. Gandrud, E. Durham, et al., "Sequential Comparisons of One-Month and Three-Month Depot Leuprolide Regimens in Central Precocious Puberty," *Journal of Clinical Endocrinology and Metabolism* (91) 2006: 1862–1867.

23. F. M. Saleh, T. Niel, and M. J. Fishman, "Treatment of Paraphilia in Young Adults with Leuprolide Acetate: A Preliminary Case Report

Series," *Journal of Forensic Science* 49 (2004): 1343–1348; J. M. Schober, P. J. Kuhn, P. G. Kovacs, J. H. Earle, P. M. Byrne, and R. A. Fries, "Leuprolide Acetate Suppresses Pedophilic Urges and Arousability," *Archives of Sexual Behavior* 34 (2005): 691–705; J. M. Schober, P. M. Byrne, and P. J. Kuhn, "Leuprolide Acetate Is a Familiar Drug That May Modify Sex-Offender Behaviour: The Urologist's Role," *BJU International* 97 (2006): 684–686.

24. H. A. Young, D. A. Geier, and M. R. Geier, "Thimerosal Exposure in Infants and Neurodevelopmental Disorders: An Assessment of Computerized Medical Records in the Vaccine Safety Datalink," *Journal of the Neurological Sciences* 271 (2008): 110–118.

25. M. R. Geier and D. A. Geier, "Thimerosal in Childhood Vaccines, Neurodevelopment Disorders, and Heart Disease in the United States," *Journal of the American Physicians and Surgeons* 8 (2003): 6–11.

26. AAP, "Study Fails to Show a Connection between Thimerosal and Autism," May 16, 2003, https://web.archive.org/web/20030604060812 /http://aap.org/profed/thimaut-may03.htm.

27. G. Harris and A. O'Connor, "On Autism's Cause, It's Parents vs. Research," *New York Times*, June 25, 2005, www.nytimes.com/2005/06 /25/science/on-autisms-cause-its-parents-vs-research.html.

28. Orac, "The Geiers Try to Patent Chemical Castration as an Autism Treatment," Respectful Insolence, April 10, 2006, https:// respectfulinsolence.com/2006/04/10/the-geiers-try-to-patent-chemi/; A. Cooper, E. M. Gopalakrishna, and D. A. Norton, "The Crystal Structure and Absolute Configuration of the 2:1 Complex between Testosterone and Mercuric Chloride," *Acta Crystallographica* B 24 (1968): 935–941.

29. G. M. Realmuto and L. A. Ruble, "Sexual Behaviors in Autism: Problems of Definition and Management," *Journal of Autism and Developmental Disorders* 29 (1999): 121–127.

30. Kathleen Seidel, "Significant Misrepresentations: Mark Geier, David Geier & the Evolution of the Lupron Protocol (Part Twelve)," Neurodiversity Weblog, November 17, 2006, http://web.archive.org/web/2007 0708153149/http://neurodiversity.com/weblog/article/116/.

31. Kathleen Seidel, "Significant Misrepresentations: Mark Geier, David Geier & the Evolution of the Lupron Protocol (Part Thirteen)," Neurodiversity Weblog, January 23, 2007, http://web.archive.org/web /20070703013255/http://neurodiversity.com/weblog/article/124/.

32. Stephen Barrett, "Maryland Medical Board Suspends Dr. Mark Geier's License," Casewatch, https://casewatch.net/board/med/geier/order .shtml. (Accessed November 10, 2018.)

33. Orac, "No, Antivaccine Quack Mark Geier Has Not Been Exonerated, but the Maryland Board of Physicians Appears to Have Screwed Up," *Respectful Insolence* (blog), February 6, 2018, https://respectfulinsolence .com/2018/02/06/antivaccine-quack-mark-geier-has-not-been-exonerated/.

34. "'What Kind of Society Do You Want to Live In?': Inside the Country Where Down Syndrome Is Disappearing" CBS News, August 14, 2017, www.cbsnews.com/news/down-syndrome-iceland/.

35. S. Sirucek, "The Parents Who Give Their Children Bleach Enemas to 'Cure' Them of Autism," Vice, March 11, 2015, www.vice.com/en_uk /article/kwxq3w/parents-are-giving-their-children-bleach-enemas-to -cure-them-of-autism-311.

36. D. Ono and L. Bartley, "'Church of Bleach': ABC News Confronts Founder of Genesis II Church," ABC7 Los Angeles, October 28, 2016, https://abc7.com/1578279/. The author finds this claim to be dubious.

37. FDA News Release, "FDA Warns Consumers of Serious Harm from Drinking Miracle Mineral Solution (MMS)," July 30, 2010, https://web .archive.org/web/20110203232945/http://www.fda.gov/NewsEvents /Newsroom/PressAnnouncements/ucm220747.htm.

38. J. Berry, "7 Children Taken from Parents during Search for 'Miracle' Treatment Chemical," KARK, January 16, 2015, www.kark.com/news /7-children-taken-from-parents-during-search-for-miracle-treatment -chemical/206833616.

39. M. Eltagouri, "A Mom Turned to a Controversial 'Treatment' for Her Daughter's Autism—Feeding Her Bleach," *Washington Post*, February 14, 2018, www.washingtonpost.com/news/to-your-health/wp/2018/02/14 /mom-accused-of-feeding-child-bleach-in-an-effort-to-cure-autism/.

40. C. Galli, R. Kreider, B. Ross, and L. Ferran, "Husband Says Fringe Church's 'Miracle Cure' Killed His Wife," ABC News, October 29, 2016, https://abcnews.go.com/US/husband-fringe-churchs-miracle-cure-killed -wife/story?id=43081647.

41. Keiligh Baker, "Mother Investigated over Using Bleach to Cure Son's Autism," *Daily Mail*, August 7, 2017, www.dailymail.co.uk/news/article -4767618/Mother-investigated-using-bleach-cure-son-s-autism.html.

42. D. A. Rossignol and L. W. Rossignol, "Hyperbaric Oxygen Therapy May Improve Symptoms in Autistic Children," *Medical Hypotheses* 67 (2006): 216–228.

43. Wake Forest University Baptist Medical Center, "Does Manganese Inhaled from the Shower Represent a Public Health Threat?" *Science Daily*, July 4, 2005, www.sciencedaily.com/releases/2005/07/050704114441 .htm.

44. G. Steinhauser, "The Nature of Navel Fluff," *Medical Hypotheses* 72 (2009): 623–625.

45. Martin Enserink, "Elsevier to Editor: Change Controversial Journal or Resign," ScienceMag.org, March 8, 2010, www.sciencemag.org/news /2010/03/elsevier-editor-change-controversial-journal-or-resign.

46. D. A. Rossignol, L. W. Rossignol, S. J. James, S. Melnyk, and E. Mumper, "The Effects of Hyperbaric Oxygen Therapy on Oxidative Stress, Inflammation, and Symptoms in Children with Autism: An Open-Label Pilot Study," *BMC Pediatrics* 2007;7: 36.

47. D. A. Rossignol, J. J. Bradstreet, K. Van Dyke, C. Schneider, S. H. Freedenfeld, N. O'Hara, et al., "Hyperbaric Oxygen Treatment in Autism Spectrum Disorders," *Medical Gas Research* 2 (2012): 16.

48. D. A. Rossignol, L. W. Rossignol, S. Smith, C. Schneider, S. Loger-quist, A. Usman, et al., "Hyperbaric Treatment for Children with Autism: A Multicenter, Randomized, Double-Blind, Controlled Trial," *BMC Pediatrics* 9 (2009): 21.

49. S. Novella, "Hyperbaric Oxygen for Autism," NeuroLogica Blog, March 16, 2009, https://theness.com/neurologicablog/index.php/hyperbaric -oxygen-for-autism/.

50. D. Granpeesheh, J. Tarbox, D. R. Dixon, A. E. Wilke, M. S. Allen, and J. J. Bradstreet, "Randomized Trial of Hyperbaric Oxygen Therapy for Children with Autism," *Research in Autism Spectrum Disorders* 4 (2010): 268–275.

51. P. Callahan, "Doctors Sued Over 'Dangerous' Autism Treatment," *Chicago Tribune*, March 4, 2010, www.chicagotribune.com/living/ct -xpm-2010-03-04-ct-met-autism-therapy-lawsuit-20100304-story.html.

52. K. Horvath, G. Stefanatos, K. N. Sokolski, R. Wachtel, L. Nabors, and J. T. Tildon, "Improved Social and Language Skills after Secretin Administration in Patients with Autistic Spectrum Disorders," *Journal of the Association of Academic Minority Physicians* 9 (1998): 9–15.

53. Steve Bunk, "Secretin Trials: A Drug That Might Help, or Hurt, Autistic Children Is Widely Prescribed but Is Just Now Being Tested," *Scientist*, June 12, 1999, www.the-scientist.com/news/secretin-trials-a-drug-that -might-help-or-hurt-autistic-children-is-widely-prescribed-but-is-just-now -being-tested-56430.

54. K. Williams, J. A. Wray, and D. M. Wheeler, "Intravenous Secretin for Autism Spectrum Disorders (ASD)," *Cochrane Database of Systematic Reviews* (2012): CD003495.

55. D. Collins, "Autistic Boy Dies during Exorcism," CBS News, August 26, 2003, www.cbsnews.com/news/autistic-boy-dies-during-exorcism/.

56. Upledger Foundation, "Autism," www.upledger.org/autism.

57. M. M. Cohen Jr., "Sutural Biology and the Correlates of Craniosynostosis," *American Journal of Medical Genetics* 47 (1993): 581–616.

58. S. E. Hartman and J. M. Norton, "Craniosacral Therapy Is Not Medicine," *Physical Therapy* 82 (2002): 1146–1147.

59. C. Green, C. W. Martin, K. Bassett, and A. Kazanjian, *A Systematic Review and Critical Appraisal of the Scientific Evidence on Craniosacral Therapy* (Centre for Reviews and Dissemination, 1999).

60. In conversation, a DO student related to me that he had been forced to train in craniosacral therapy against his protests that it was not evidence based. His ability to sense "primary respiration" disappeared

when he asked the patient to hold his breath. Most likely "primary respiration" is a misattributed feeling of actual respiration.

61. A. Fasano and C. Catassi, "Clinical Practice: Celiac Disease," *New England Journal of Medicine* 367 (2012): 2419–2426.

62. Autistic Self Advocacy Network, "Statement on Autism Speaks Board Appointments," December 2015, https://autisticadvocacy.org/2015/12 /statement-on-autism-speaks-board-appointments/.

63. thecaffeinatedautistic, "Why I Am against Autism Speaks (and You Should Be, Too)," The Caffeinated Autistic March 5, 2013, https:// thecaffeinatedautistic.wordpress.com/2013/03/05/why-i-am-against -autism-speaks-and-you-should-be-too-2/.

64. D. Mitchell, "Autism Activist Says It's Time to Acknowledge There's No Autism-Vaccine Link," AAFP, August 4, 2009, www.aafp.org/news /vaccine/20090804singerinterview.html.

65. "What Causes Autism?" Autism Speaks, www.autismspeaks.org/what -causes-autism.

66. L. Berrington, "A Reporter's Guide to the Autism Speaks Debacle," *Psychology Today*, November 14, 2013, www.psychologytoday.com/blog /aspergers-alive/201311/reporters-guide-the-autism-speaks-debacle.

Chapter 14

1. Adolf Hitler, in his rise to power, used the phrase "lying press"; however, "fake news" is more apropos in the current political landscape.

2. D. J. J. Lazer, M. A. Baum, Y. Benkler, A. J. Berinsky, K. M. Greenhill, F. Menczer, et al., "The Science of Fake News," *Science* 359 (2018): 1094–1096.

3. Life has not yet been discovered on the moon. See B. Thornton, "The Moon Hoax: Debates about Ethics in 1835 New York Newspapers," *Journal of Mass Media Ethics* 15 (2000): 89–100.

4. J. Gottfried and E. Shearer, "News Use across Social Media Platforms 2016," Pew Research Center's Journalism Project, May 26, 2016, www

.journalism.org/2016/05/26/news-use-across-social-media-platforms
-2016/.

5. H. Allcott and M. Gentzkow, "Social Media and Fake News in the
2016 Election," *Journal of Economic Perspectives* 31 (2017): 211–236.

6. S. Vosoughi, D. Roy, and S. Aral, "The Spread of True and False News
Online," *Science* 359 (2018): 1146–1151.

7. C. Stempel, T. Hargrove, and G. H. Stempel, "Media Use, Social Structure, and Belief in 9/11 Conspiracy Theories," *Journalism and Mass Communication Quarterly* 84 (2007): 353–372.

8. S. Fox, "The Social Life of Health Information, 2011," Pew Research
Center: Internet, Science & Tech, May 12, 2011, www.pewinternet.org
/2011/05/12/the-social-life-of-health-information-2011/.

9. D. Jolley and K. M. Douglas, "The Effects of Anti-Vaccine Conspiracy
Theories on Vaccination Intentions," *PLoS One* 9 (2014): e89177.

10. Public Policy Polling, "Press Release: Democrats and Republicans
Differ on Conspiracy Theory Beliefs," April 2, 2013, www.publicpolicy
polling.com/wp-content/uploads/2017/09/PPP_Release_National_Con
spiracyTheories_040213.pdf.

11. P. Davies, S. Chapman, and J. Leask, "Antivaccination Activists on
the World Wide Web," *Archives of Disease in Childhood* 87 (2002): 22–25.

12. P. Kortum, C. Edwards, R. Richards-Kortum, "The Impact of Inaccurate Internet Health Information in a Secondary School Learning
Environment," *Journal of Medical Internet Research* 10 (2008): e17.

13. The naturalistic fallacy occurs when something is assumed to be good
because it exists in nature. In reality, many bad or dangerous things exist
in nature that can be harmful to human health and well-being, such as
disease-causing microorganisms and disembowelment-causing bears.

14. S. J. Bean, "Emerging and Continuing Trends in Vaccine Opposition
Website Content," *Vaccine* 29 (2011): 1874–1880.

15. A. Kata, "A Postmodern Pandora's Box: Anti-Vaccination Misinformation on the Internet," *Vaccine* 28 (2010): 1709–1716.

16. Some of the cultured cells used in the production of certain live or inactivated virus vaccines are derived from the lungs of an aborted fetus; however, the phrasing "aborted fetal tissue" is misleading. No abortion occurred specifically to produce the cells, and the cells have been growing in culture for many decades.

17. N. Seeman, A. Ing, and C. Rizo, "Assessing and Responding in Real Time to Online Anti-Vaccine Sentiment during a Flu Pandemic," *Healthcare Quarterly* 13 (2010), Spec No: 8–15.

18. G. A. Poland and R. J. Jacobson, "The Age-Old Struggle against the Antivaccinationists," *New England Journal of Medicine* 364 (2011): 97–99.

19. J. Keelan, V. Pavri-Garcia, G. Tomlinson, and K. Wilson, "YouTube as a Source of Information on Immunization: A Content Analysis," *JAMA* 298 (2007): 2482–2484.

20. R. Briones, X. Nan, K. Madden, and L. Waks, "When Vaccines Go Viral: An Analysis of HPV Vaccine Coverage on YouTube," *Health Communication* 27 (2012): 478–485.

21. L. G. van Hilten, "Anti-Vaccine Posts Are Going 'Under the Radar' on Pinterest," Elsevier Connect, February 1, 2016, www.elsevier.com /connect/anti-vaccine-posts-are-going-under-the-radar-on-pinterest; J. P. D. Guidry, K. Carlyle, M. Messner, and Y. Jin, "On Pins and Needles: How Vaccines Are Portrayed on Pinterest," *Vaccine* 33 (2015): 5051–5056.

22. J. Horwitz, "Facebook Pledged Crackdown on Vaccine Misinformation. Then Not Much Happened," *WSJ Online*, May 30, 2019, www.wsj .com/articles/facebook-pledged-crackdown-on-vaccine-misinformation -then-not-much-happened-11559243847.

23. Merriam-Webster.com, s.v. "meme," www.merriam-webster.com /dictionary/meme.

24. W. Sommer, "Facebook Won't Stop Dangerous Anti-Vaccine Hoaxes from Spreading," *The Daily Beast*, July 25, 2018, www.thedailybeast.com /facebook-wont-stop-dangerous-anti-vaccine-hoaxes-from-spreading.

25. M. Amith and C. Tao, "Representing Vaccine Misinformation Using Ontologies," *Journal of Biomedical Semantics* 9 (2018): 22.

26. K. Roose, "Facebook Banned InfoWars. Now What?" *New York Times*, August 10, 2018, www.nytimes.com/2018/08/10/technology/face book-banned-infowars-now-what.html.

27. K. Weill, "Facebook Removes Conspiracy Site Natural News," *The Daily Beast*, June 10, 2019 www.thedailybeast.com/facebook-removes -conspiracy-site-natural-news.

28. L. Matsakis, Z. Karabell, K. Finley, and T. Simonite, "Facebook Will Crack Down on Anti-Vaccine Content," *Wired*, March 7, 2019, www .wired.com/story/facebook-anti-vaccine-crack-down/.

29. "Email Marketer Mailchimp Bans Anti-Vaccination Content," NBC News, June 13 2019, www.nbcnews.com/tech/tech-news/email -marketer-mailchimp-bans-anti-vaccination-content-n1017221.

30. K. Ho, "Defending a Culture of Free Speech," *Harvard Political Review*, April 9, 2017, http://harvardpolitics.com/harvard/defending-culture-free -speech/.

31. S. J. Ceci and W. M. Williams, "Who Decides What Is Acceptable Speech on Campus? Why Restricting Free Speech Is Not the Answer," *Perspectives on Psychological Science* 13 (2018): 299–323.

32. A. Venkatraman, D. Mukhija, N. Kumar, and S. J. S. Nagpal, "Zika Virus Misinformation on the Internet," *Travel Medicine and Infectious Diseases* 14 (2016): 421–422.

33. B. Seymour, R. Getman, A. Saraf, L. H. Zhang, and E. Kalenderian, "When Advocacy Obscures Accuracy Online: Digital Pandemics of Public Health Misinformation through an Antifluoride Case Study," *American Journal of Public Health* 105 (2015): 517–523.

34. R. F. Baumeister, L. Zhang, and K. D. Vohs, "Gossip as Cultural Learning," *Review of General Psychology* 8 (2004): 111–121.

35. Climate change is real and caused in large part by human activity. D. M. Kahan, E. Peters, M. Wittlin, P. Slovic, L. L. Ouellette, D. Braman,

et al., "The Polarizing Impact of Science Literacy and Numeracy on Perceived Climate Change Risks," *Nature Climate Change* 2 (2012): 732.

36. C. G. Lord, L. Ross, and M. R. Lepper, "Biased Assimilation and Attitude Polarization: The Effects of Prior Theories on Subsequently Considered Evidence," *Journal of Personality and Social Psychology* 37 (1979): 2098–2109.

37. M. J. Metzger, A. J. Flanagin, and R. B. Medders, "Social and Heuristic Approaches to Credibility Evaluation Online," *Journal of Communication* 60 (2010): 413–439.

38. D. M. Kahan, D. Braman, G. L. Cohen, J. Gastil, and P. Slovic, "Who Fears the HPV Vaccine, Who Doesn't, and Why? An Experimental Study of the Mechanisms of Cultural Cognition," *Law and Human Behavior* 34 (2010): 501–516.

39. A. H. Hastorf and H. Cantril, "They Saw a Game: A Case Study," *Journal of Abnormal Psychology* 49 (1954): 129–134.

40. J. Kruger and D. Dunning, "Unskilled and Unaware of It: How Difficulties in Recognizing One's Own Incompetence Lead to Inflated Self-Assessments," *Journal of Personality and Social Psychology* 77 (1999): 1121–1134.

41. J. Krueger and R. A. Mueller, "Unskilled, Unaware, or Both? The Better-Than-Average Heuristic and Statistical Regression Predict Errors in Estimates of Own Performance," *Journal of Personality and Social Psychology* 82 (2002): 180–188.

42. M. Krajc and A. Ortmann, "Are the Unskilled Really That Unaware? An Alternative Explanation," *Journal of Economic Psychology* 29 (2008): 724–738.

43. J. Ehrlinger, T. Gilovich, and L. Ross, "Peering into the Bias Blind Spot: People's Assessments of Bias in Themselves and Others," *Personality and Social Psychology Bulletin* 31 (2005): 680–692; E. Pronin, D. Y. Lin, and L. Ross, "The Bias Blind Spot: Perceptions of Bias in Self versus Others," *Personality and Social Psychology Bulletin* 28 (2002): 369–381.

44. E. Pronin, T. Gilovich, and L. Ross, "Objectivity in the Eye of the Beholder: Divergent Perceptions of Bias in Self versus Others," *Psychological Review* 111 (2004): 781–799.

45. N. C. Bakke, "Robert's Rules of Order," in *Dicta* (HeinOnline, 1944), 85.

46. J. Allgaier, S. Dunwoody, D. Brossard, Y.-Y. Lo, and H. P. Peters, "Journalism and Social Media as Means of Observing the Contexts of Science," *Bioscience* 63 (2013): 284–287.

47. C. O'Connor, G. Rees, and H. Joffe, "Neuroscience in the Public Sphere," *Neuron* 74 (2012): 220–226.

48. H. M. Bik and M. C. Goldstein, "An Introduction to Social Media for Scientists," *PLoS Biology* 11 (2013): e1001535.

49. A. Dudo, D. Brossard, J. Shanahan, D. A. Scheufele, M. Morgan, and N. Signorielli, "Science on Television in the 21st Century: Recent Trends in Portrayals and Their Contributions to Public Attitudes toward Science," *Communication Research* 38 (2011): 754–777.

50. L. Y.-F. Su, M. A. Cacciatore, D. A. Scheufele, D. Brossard, and M. A. Xenos, "Inequalities in Scientific Understanding: Differentiating between Factual and Perceived Knowledge Gaps," *Science Communication* 36 (2014): 352–378.

51. C. Betsch, F. Renkewitz, T. Betsch, and C. Ulshöfer, "The Influence of Vaccine-Critical Websites on Perceiving Vaccination Risks," *Journal of Health Psychology* 15 (2010): 446–455.

52. C. Betsch and F. Renkewitz, "Long-term Effects of an Information Search on Vaccine-Critical Internet Sites," *Prävention* 32 (2009): 125–128.

53. "The Case for a 'Deficit Model' of Science Communication," SciDev .net, June 27, 2005, www.scidev.net/index.cfm?originalUrl=/global /communication/editorials/the-case-for-a-deficit-model-of-science -communic.html&.

54. N. Allum, P. Sturgis, D. Tabourazi, and I. Brunton-Smith, "Science Knowledge and Attitudes across Cultures: A Meta-analysis," *Public Understanding of Science* 17 (2008): 35–54.

55. S. L. Popkin, *The Reasoning Voter: Communication and Persuasion in Presidential Campaigns* (Chicago: University of Chicago Press, 1994).

56. D. A. Scheufele, "Messages and Heuristics: How Audiences Form Attitudes about Emerging Technologies," in *Engaging Science: Thoughts, Deeds, Analysis and Action*, ed. J. Turney (London: The Wellcome Trust, 2006).

57. D. A. Scheufele, "Communicating Science in Social Settings," *Proceedings of the National Academy of Sciences* 110, suppl. 3 (2013): 14040–14047.

Chapter 15

1. B. M. Staw, "The Escalation of Commitment to Course of Action," *Academy of Management Review* 6, no. 4 (1981): 577–587, www.gwern.net/docs/sunkcosts/1981-staw.pdf.

2. R. L. Schaumberg and S. S. Wiltermuth, "Desire for a Positive Moral Self-Regard Exacerbates Escalation of Commitment to Initiatives with Prosocial Aims," *Organizational Behavior and Human Decision Processes* 123 (2014): 110–123.

3. E. H. Kessler, *Encyclopedia of Management Theory* (Thousand Oaks, CA: SAGE, 2013).

4. B. Dietz-Uhler, "The Escalation of Commitment in Political Decision-Making Groups: A Social Identity Approach," *European Journal of Social Psychology* 26 (1996): 611–629.

5. D. G. Myers and H. Lamm, "The Polarizing Effect of Group Discussion," *American Scientist* 63 (1975): 297–303.

6. S. Yardi and D. Boyd, "Dynamic Debates: An Analysis of Group Polarization over Time on Twitter," *Bulletin of Science, Technology & Society* 30 (2010): 316–327.

Chapter 16

1. G. Pelčić, S. Karačić, G. L. Mikirtichan, O. I. Kubar, G. J. Leavitt, M. Cheng-Tek Tai, et al. "Religious Exception for Vaccination or Religious

Excuses for Avoiding Vaccination," *Croatian Medical Journal* 57 (2016): 516–521.

2. J. D. Grabenstein, "What the World's Religions Teach, Applied to Vaccines and Immune Globulins," *Vaccine* 31 (2013): 2011–2023.

3. W. L. M. Ruijs, J. L. A. Hautvast, S. Kerrar, K. van der Velden, and M. E. J. L. Hulscher, "The Role of Religious Leaders in Promoting Acceptance of Vaccination within a Minority Group: A Qualitative Study," *BMC Public Health* 13 (2013): 511.

4. A. Imdad, B. Tserenpuntsag, D. S. Blog, N. A. Halsey, D. E. Easton, and J. Shaw, "Religious Exemptions for Immunization and Risk of Pertussis in New York State, 2000–2011," *Pediatrics* 132 (2013): 37–43.

5. R. C. Shelton, A. C. Snavely, M. De Jesus, M. D. Othus, and J. D. Allen, "HPV Vaccine Decision-Making and Acceptance: Does Religion Play a Role?" *Journal of Religion and Health* 52 (2013): 1120–1130.

6. W. L. M. Ruijs, J. L. A. Hautvast, G. van IJzendoorn, W. J. C. van Ansem, G. Elwyn, K. van der Velden, et al., "How Healthcare Professionals Respond to Parents with Religious Objections to Vaccination: A Qualitative Study," *BMC Health Services Research* 12 (2012): 231.

7. A. Ahmed, K. S. Lee, A. Bukhsh, Y. M. Al-Worafi, M. M. R. Sarker, L. C. Ming, et al. "Outbreak of Vaccine-Preventable Diseases in Muslim Majority Countries," *Journal of Infection and Public Health* 11 (2018): 153–155.

8. The dates of the hajj depend on the lunar calendar and therefore do not fall on identical dates of the Gregorian calendar each year.

9. G. Y. Ahmed, H. H. Balkhy, S. Bafaqeer, B. Al-Jasir, and A. Althaqafi, "Acceptance and Adverse Effects of H1N1 Vaccinations among a Cohort of National Guard Health Care Workers during the 2009 Hajj Season," *BMC Research Notes* 4 (2011): 61.

10. Q. A. Ahmed, Y. M. Arabi, Z. A. Memish, "Health Risks at the Hajj," *Lancet* 367 (2006): 1008–1015.

11. D. G. McNeil Jr., "Saudis Try to Head Off Swine Flu Fears before Hajj," *New York Times*, October 29, 2009, www.nytimes.com/2009/10/30/world/middleeast/30flu.html.

12. A. Mullaney and S. A. Hassan, "He Led the CIA to bin Laden—and Unwittingly Fueled a Vaccine Backlash," *National Geographic*, February 27, 2015, https://news.nationalgeographic.com/2015/02/150227-polio-pakistan-vaccination-taliban-osama-bin-laden/.

13. "How the CIA's Fake Vaccination Campaign Endangers Us All," *Scientific American*, May 1, 2013, www.scientificamerican.com/article/how-cia-fake-vaccination-campaign-endangers-us-all/.

14. D. Walsh and D. G. McNeil Jr., "Female Vaccination Workers, Essential in Pakistan, Become Prey," *New York Times*, December 20, 2012, www.nytimes.com/2012/12/21/world/asia/un-halts-vaccine-work-in-pakistan-after-more-killings.html.

15. D. G. McNeil Jr., "Gunmen Kill Nigerian Polio Vaccine Workers in Echo of Pakistan Attacks," *New York Times*, February 9, 2013, www.nytimes.com/2013/02/09/world/africa/in-nigeria-polio-vaccine-workers-are-killed-by-gunmen.html.

16. "Nigeria Restarts Polio Campaign," BBC News, July 31, 2004, http://news.bbc.co.uk/2/hi/health/3942349.stm.

17. C. Chen, "Rebellion against the Polio Vaccine in Nigeria: Implications for Humanitarian Policy," *African Health Sciences* 4 (2004): 205–207.

18. S. Saifi and D. Andone, "Two Polio Workers Killed in Pakistan," CNN, March 18, 2018, www.cnn.com/2018/03/18/world/polio-workers-killed-pakistan/index.html.

19. "Race Is On to Create 'Halal' Measles Vaccine," *Daily Telegraph*, August 22, 2018, www.telegraph.co.uk/news/0/race-create-halal-measles-vaccine/.

20. CDC, Travelers' Health, "Measles in Indonesia: Watch-Level 1, Practice Usual Precautions," wwwnc.cdc.gov/travel/notices/watch/measles-indonesia.

21. OU Staff, "Statement on Vaccinations from the OU and Rabbinical Council of America," November 14, 2018, www.ou.org/news/statement-vaccinations-ou-rabbinical-council-america/.

22. M. Andrews, "Why Measles Hits So Hard within N.Y. Orthodox Jewish Community," Kaiser Health News, March 11, 2019, https://khn.org/news /why-measles-hits-so-hard-within-n-y-orthodox-jewish-community/.

23. A. Pink and A. Feldman, "We Read the Guide Fueling Ultra-Orthodox Fears of Pig Blood in Measles Vaccines," *Forward*, April 11, 2019, https:// forward.com/news/national/422354/hasidic-measles-outbreak-peach -handbook/.

24. Gwynne Hogan, "Ultra-Orthodox Brooklyn Residents Protest Anti-Vax Symposium," *Gothamist*, June 5, 2019, http://gothamist.com/2019 /06/05/ultra-orthodox_vaccination_protest.php.

25. J. D. Grabenstein, "What the World's Religions Teach, Applied to Vaccines and Immune Globulins," *Vaccine* 31 (2013): 2011–2023.

26. Y. S. Yoder and M. S. Dworkin, "Vaccination Usage among an Old-Order Amish Community in Illinois," *Pediatric Infectious Disease Journal* 25 (2006): 1182–1183.

27. O. K. Wenger, M. D. McManus, J. R. Bower, and D. L. Langkamp, "Underimmunization in Ohio's Amish: Parental Fears Are a Greater Obstacle Than Access to Care," *Pediatrics* 128 (2011): 79–85.

28. CDC, "Epidemiologic Notes and Reports Multiple Measles Outbreaks on College Campuses—Ohio, Massachusetts, Illinois," March 15, 1985, www.cdc.gov/mmwr/preview/mmwrhtml/00000500.htm.

29. CDC, "Measles in a Population with Religious Exemption to Vaccination—Colorado," November 29, 1985, www.cdc.gov/mmwr /preview/mmwrhtml/00000644.htm.

30. CDC, "Outbreak of Measles among Christian Science Students—Missouri and Illinois, 1994," July 1, 1994, www.cdc.gov/mmwr/preview /mmwrhtml/00031788.htm.

31. N. A. Talbot, "The Position of the Christian Science Church," *New England Journal of Medicine* 309 (1983): 1641–1644.

32. "Scientology Silent Birth: 'It's a Natural Thing': The Rev. John Carmichael of the Church of Scientology Explains Why His Religion

Frowns on Talking during Labor and Delivery," Beliefnet.com, www
.beliefnet.com/Faiths/Scientology/Scientology-Silent-Birth-Its-A-Natural
-Thing.aspx?p=4.

33. A. Memon, "Cross-border Lessons in Saving Lives," *Hindu*, September 20, 2012, www.thehindu.com/todays-paper/tp-opinion/crossborder
-lessons-in-saving-lives/article3916454.ece.

34. "Don't Use 'Mormon' or 'LDS' as Church Name, President Says,"
NBC News, August 16, 2018, www.nbcnews.com/news/us-news/don-t
-use-mormon-or-lds-church-name-president-says-n901491.

35. The Church of Jesus Christ of Latter-Day Saints, "Immunize Children, Leaders Urge," July 1978, www.lds.org/liahona/1978/07/immunize
-children-leaders-urge?lang=eng.

36. The Church of Jesus Christ of Latter-Day Saints, "Immunizations—a
Reminder," July 1985, www.lds.org/ensign/1985/07/random-sampler
/immunizations-a-reminder?lang=eng.

37. The Church of Jesus Christ of Latter-Day Saints, "Church Makes
Immunizations an Official Initiative, Provides Social Mobilization,"
June 13, 2012, www.lds.org/church/news/church-makes-immunizations
-an-official-initiative-provides-social-mobilization?lang=eng&_r=1.

38. The author's discussions with TST members suggest that the primary intent of this tenet is to uphold bodily autonomy, particularly as it
applies to reproductive rights.

39. "Parents Fake Religion to Avoid Vaccines," CBS News, October 17,
2007, www.cbsnews.com/news/parents-fake-religion-to-avoid-vaccines/.

40. However, proving that one holds a particular religious belief is not
generally possible.

41. "From the Danbury Baptist Association," in *The Papers of Thomas
Jefferson*, vol. 35: *1 August to 30 November 1801* (Princeton, NJ: Princeton
University Press, 2008), 407–409, https://jeffersonpapers.princeton.edu
/selected-documents/danbury-baptist-association.

Chapter 17

1. R. Hofstadter, A. Cudi, F. Turner, B. Lopez, M. Houellebecq, J. Cullen, et al., "The Paranoid Style in American Politics," *Harper's*, November 1964, https://harpers.org/archive/1964/11/the-paranoid-style-in-american-politics/.

2. Although the profit motive of lawyers suing large pharmaceutical companies is rarely discussed in such detail.

3. S. Kaplan, G. B. Calkins, S. J. Sarnoff, and N. Lawrence Dalling, "Hypodermic Injection Device Having Means for Varying the Medicament Capacity Thereof," US Patent 4031893, 1977, https://patentimages.storage.googleapis.com/8b/f5/07/91f9322d3897b4/US4031893.pdf.

4. R. Rubin, "EpiPen Price Hike Comes under Scrutiny," *Lancet* 388 (2016): 1266.

5. "Big Pharma Ushers in New Year by Raising Prices of More Than 1,000 Drugs," CBS News, January 2, 2019, www.cbsnews.com/news/drug-prices-oxycontin-predaxa-purdue-pharmaceuticals-boehringer-ingelheim/?fbclid=IwAR1Jy3go6-5SfvuIau-j0MqajWSF-aeFUfwilStEvCiPUXg6f-EemkXZ2PQ.

6. J. Lexchin, "Pharmaceutical Company Spending on Research and Development and Promotion in Canada, 2013–2016: A Cohort Analysis," *Journal of Pharmaceutical Policy and Practice* 11 (2018): 5.

7. D. Mukherjee, S. E. Nissen, and E. J. Topol, "Risk of Cardiovascular Events associated with Selective COX-2 Inhibitors," *JAMA* 286 (2001): 954–959.

8. E. J. Topol, "Failing the Public Health—Rofecoxib, Merck, and the FDA," *New England Journal of Medicine* 351 (2004): 1707–1709.

9. Anna Wilde Mathews and Barbara Martinez, "E-mails Suggest Merck Knew Vioxx's Dangers at Early Stage," WSJ.com, November 1, 2004, www.wsj.com/articles/SB109926864290160719.

10. R. Horton, "Vioxx, the Implosion of Merck, and Aftershocks at the FDA," *Lancet* 364 (2004) 1995–1996.

11. K. J. Winstein, "Top Pain Scientist Fabricated Data in Studies, Hospital Says," WSJ.com, March 11, 2009, www.wsj.com/articles/SB123 672510903888207.

12. Lydia Saad, "Restaurants Again Voted Most Popular U.S. Industry," Gallup.com, August 15, 2016, https://news.gallup.com/poll/194570/rest aurants-again-voted-popular-industry.aspx.

13. Z. Harel, S. Harel, R.Wald, M. Mamdani, and C. M. Bell, "The Frequency and Characteristics of Dietary Supplement Recalls in the United States," *JAMA Internal Medicine* 173 (2013): 926–928.

14. "Dietary Supplements Market Size Worth $278.02 Billion by 2024," May 2019, www.grandviewresearch.com/press-release/global-dietary -supplements-market.

15. R. Blaskiewicz, "The Big Pharma Conspiracy Theory," *Medical Writing* 22 (2013): 259–261.

16. S. Clarke, "Conspiracy Theories and Conspiracy Theorizing," *Philosophy of the Social Sciences* 32 (2002): 131–150.

17. J. A. Whitson and A. D. Galinsky, "Lacking Control Increases Illusory Pattern Perception," *Science* 322 (2008): 115–117.

18. See anyone who responds to this book by calling the author a shill for Big Pharma.

19. J. A. Whitson and A. D. Galinsky, "Lacking Control Increases Illusory Pattern Perception," *Science* 322 (2008): 115–117.

20. R. Brotherton and C. French, "Belief in Conspiracy Theories and Susceptibility to the Conjunction Fallacy," *Applied Cognitive Psychology* 28 (2014): 238–248; K. M. Douglas and A. C. Leite, "Suspicion in the Workplace: Organizational Conspiracy Theories and Work-Related Outcomes," *British Journal of Psychology* 108 (2017): 486–506.

21. The most famous example of the conjunction fallacy is the Linda Problem. When Linda was a student, she was active in social-justice causes, cared deeply about animal welfare, and studied zoology. Which is more likely: that Linda works at a bank or that Linda works at a bank and

is a vegetarian? We might be tempted to choose the latter, but in fact the former is more likely. Let's say there is a 20 percent (0.2) probability that Linda works at a bank and a 99 percent (0.99) probability that Linda is a vegetarian. The probability that both are true is (0.2*0.99=0.198). Because 19.8 percent is less than 20 percent, it is less probable that Linda is a banker and a vegetarian than that she is just a banker.

22. K. M. Douglas and A. C. Leite, "Suspicion in the Workplace: Organizational Conspiracy Theories and Work-Related Outcomes," *British Journal of Psychology* 108 (2017): 486–506.

23. K. R. Popper, "The Conspiracy Theory of Society," www3.canyons .edu/faculty/marianaj/Popper.pdf. (Accessed November 15, 2019.)

24. C. Pigden, "Popper Revisited, or What Is Wrong With Conspiracy Theories?" *Philosophy of the Social Sciences* 25 (1995): 3–34.

25. R. Blaskiewicz, "The Big Pharma Conspiracy Theory," *Medical Writing* 22 (2013): 259–261.

26. C. L. Ventola, "The Antibiotic Resistance Crisis: Part 1: Causes and Threats," *P&T Community* 40 (2015): 277–283.

27. IMS Health Market Prognosis, "Total Unaudited and Audited Global Pharmaceutical Market by Region," www.skepticalraptor.com/blog /wp-content/uploads/2013/05/Regional_Pharma_Market_by_Spend ing_2011-2016.pdf. (Last accessed January 17, 2020.)

28. Miloud Kaddar, "Global Vaccine Market Future and Trends," World Health Organization, www.skepticalraptor.com/blog/wp-content/uploads /2013/05/Vaccine-Market-Value.pdf. (Last accessed January 17, 2020.)

29. P. A. Rochon, J. H. Gurwitz, R. W. Simms, P. R. Fortin, D. T. Felson, K. L. Minaker, et al., "A Study of Manufacturer-Supported Trials of Nonsteroidal Anti-inflammatory Drugs in the Treatment of Arthritis," *Archives of Internal Medicine* 154 (1994): 157–163.

30. M. K. Cho and L. A. Bero, "The Quality of Drug Studies Published in Symposium Proceedings," *Annals of Internal Medicine* 124 (1996): 485–489.

31. M. Friedberg, B. Saffran, T. J. Stinson, W. Nelson, and C. L. Bennett, "Evaluation of Conflict of Interest in Economic Analyses of New Drugs Used in Oncology," *JAMA* 282 (1999): 1453–1457.

32. Technically, the uncertainty principle refers to the enrollment of an individual patient in a clinical trial, while clinical equipoise refers to the overall uncertainty of the medical profession as to which treatment is best. B. Djulbegovic, M. Lacevic, A. Cantor, K. K. Fields, C. L. Bennett, J. R. Adams, et al., "The Uncertainty Principle and Industry-Sponsored Research," *Lancet* 356 (2000): 635–638.

33. J. M. Taber, B. Leyva, and A. Persoskie, "Why Do People Avoid Medical Care? A Qualitative Study Using National Data," *Journal of General Internal Medicine* 30 (2015): 290–297.

34. F. Loeffler, *Untersuchungen über die Bedeutung der Mikroorganismen für die Entstehung der Diphtherie beim Menschen, bei der Taube und beim Kalbe* (1884).

35. R. E. DeHovitz, "The 1901 St. Louis Incident: The First Modern Medical Disaster," *Pediatrics* 133 (2014): 964–965.

36. US Food and Drug Administration, "Charter of the Vaccines and Related Biological Products Advisory Committee," last updated January 2, 2018, www.fda.gov/AdvisoryCommittees/CommitteesMeetingMaterials/BloodVaccinesandOtherBiologics/VaccinesandRelatedBiologicalProductsAdvisoryCommittee/ucm129571.htm.

37. US Food and Drug Administration, Office of the Commissioner, Applying for Membership on FDA Advisory Committees, www.fda.gov/AdvisoryCommittees/AboutAdvisoryCommittees/CommitteeMembership/ApplyingforMembership/.

38. US Department of Health and Human Services, "Vaccine Types," www.vaccines.gov/basics/types/index.html.

39. D. Lowe, "A New Look at Clinical Success Rates," *Pipeline* (blog), February 2, 2018, https://blogs.sciencemag.org/pipeline/archives/2018/02/02/a-new-look-at-clinical-success-rates.

40. National Vaccine Advisory Committee, "United States Vaccine Research: A Delicate Fabric of Public and Private Collaboration," *Pediatrics* 100 (1997): 1015–1020.

Chapter 18

1. "'Anti-vax' Movement Blamed for 30 Per Cent Jump in Measles Cases Worldwide," SBS News, November 30, 2018, www.sbs.com.au/news /anti-vax-movement-blamed-for-30-per-cent-jump-in-measles-cases -worldwide.

2. World Health Organization, "Measles Cases Spike Globally due to Gaps in Vaccination Coverage," November 29, 2018, www.who.int /news-room/detail/29-11-2018-measles-cases-spike-globally-due-to-gaps -in-vaccination-coverage.

3. L. Wamsley, "Chickenpox Outbreak Hits N.C. Private School with Low Vaccination Rates," NPR, November 20, 2018, www.npr.org/2018 /11/20/669644191/chickenpox-outbreak-hits-n-c-private-school-with -low-vaccination-rates.

4. M. Smith, A. Daniel, and R. Murphy, "See Vaccine Exemptions in Texas by School District," *Texas Tribune*, February 5, 2015, www.texastribune .org/2015/02/05/school-vaccine-exemptions-high-pockets-texas/.

5. "Vermont Schools Report Low Vaccination Rates," *Burlington Free Press*, February 5, 2015, www.burlingtonfreepress.com/story/news/local /2015/02/05/vermont-schools-vaccination-rates/22945035/.

6. G. Yee, "Waldorf School in Belmont Heights Reports Low Vaccination Rate," *Press Telegram*, January 24, 2015, www.presstelegram.com /health/20150124/waldorf-school-in-belmont-heights-reports-low -vaccination-rate.

7. G. Balk, "Vaccine Exemptions Exceed 10% at Dozens of Seattle-Area Schools," *Seattle Times*, February 6, 2015, http://blogs.seattletimes.com /fyi-guy/2015/02/04/vaccine-exemptions-exceed-10-at-dozens-of-seattle -area-schools/.

8. R. L. Goldblatt, "Rockland Measles Outbreak: New Vaccine Clinic at Palisades Center, 91 Cases Reported," *Rockland/Westchester Journal News*, December 6, 2018, www.lohud.com/story/news/local/rockland /west-nyack/2018/12/06/rockland-measles-outbreak-new-vaccine-clinic -palisades-center/2225136002/.

9. Tamar Pileggi, "Vaccination Campaign Launched in Orthodox Neighborhoods amid Measles Outbreak," *Times of Israel*, November 4, 2018, www.timesofisrael.com/vaccination-campaign-launched-in -orthodox-neighborhoods-amid-measles-outbreak/.

10. Z. Kmietowicz, "Measles: Europe Sees Record Number of Cases and 37 Deaths So Far This Year," *BMJ* 362 (2018): k3596.

11. K. Johnson, "'A Match into a Can of Gasoline': Measles Outbreak Now an Emergency in Washington State," *New York Times*, February 6, 2019, www.nytimes.com/2019/02/06/us/measles-outbreak.html.

12. F. M. Guerra, S. Bolotin, G. Lim, J. Heffernan, S. L. Deeks, Y. Li, et al., "The Basic Reproduction Number (R0) of Measles: A Systematic Review," *Lancet Infectious Diseases* 17 (2017): e420–e428.

13. CDC, "What You Should Know for the 2017–2018 Influenza Season," November 2, 2018, www.cdc.gov/flu/about/season/flu-season -2017-2018.htm.

14. D. G. McNeil Jr., "Over 80,000 Americans Died of Flu Last Winter, Highest Toll in Years," *New York Times*, October 1, 2018, www.nytimes .com/2018/10/01/health/flu-deaths-vaccine.html.

15. Nick Sloan and Caroline Sweeney, "Billboard with 'Vaccines Can Kill' Message Goes Up in Kansas City," KCTV5, September 25, 2018, www.kctv5.com/news/billboard-with-vaccines-can-kill-message-goes-up -in-kansas/article_f428826c-c10c-11e8-9401-3730f9178bec.html.

16. C. Domonoske, "Texas Nurse Loses Job after Apparently Posting about Patient in Anti-Vaxxer Group," NPR, August 29, 2018, www .npr.org/2018/08/29/642937977/texas-nurse-loses-job-after-apparently -posting-about-patient-in-anti-vaxxer-grou.

17. F. De Benedetti, "How the Anti-vaxxers Are Winning in Italy," *Independent*, September 28, 2018, www.independent.co.uk/news/world/europe /anti-vaxxers-italy-vaccine-measles-epidemic-europe-us-vaccination -global-health-security-agenda-a8560021.html.

18. "Italy's Populist Coalition Renounces Anti-Vaccination Stance amid Measles 'Emergency,'" *Daily Telegraph*, November 15, 2018, www .telegraph.co.uk/news/2018/11/15/italys-populist-coalition-renounces -anti-vaccination-stance/.

19. "Italy's Coalition Spreads Confusion over Vaccinations by Sacking Commission of Health Experts," *Daily Telegraph*, December 5, 2018, www .telegraph.co.uk/news/2018/12/05/italys-coalition-spreads-confusion -vaccinations-sacking-commission/.

20. R. Picheta, "German Government Backs Mandatory Vaccinations for All Schoolchildren," CNN, July 17, 2019, www.cnn.com/2019/07/17 /health/germany-measles-mandatory-vaccine-scli-intl/index.html.

21. Global Biodefense Staff, "The State of the Antivaccine Movement in the United States," June 28, 2018, https://globalbiodefense.com/2018 /06/28/the-state-of-the-antivaccine-movement-in-the-united-states/.

22. B. Baumgaertner, J. E. Carlisle, and F. Justwan, "The Influence of Political Ideology and Trust on Willingness to Vaccinate," *PLoS One* 13 (2018): e0191728.

Chapter 19

1. B. Nyhan, J. Reifler, S. Richey, and G. L. Freed, "Effective Messages in Vaccine Promotion: A Randomized Trial," *Pediatrics* 133 (2014): e835–842.

2. L. Gillespie, C. W. Hicks, M. Santana, S. E. Worley, D. A. Banas, S. Holmes, et al., "The Acceptability of Human Papillomavirus Vaccine among Parents and Guardians of Newborn to 10-Year-Old Children," *Journal of Pediatric and Adolescent Gynecology* 24 (2011): 66–70.

3. E. W. Clayton, G. B. Hickson, and C. S. Miller, "Parents' Responses to Vaccine Information Pamphlets," *Pediatrics* 93 (1994): 369–372.

268 Notes

4. S. S. C. Chan, T. H. Cheung, W. K. Lo, and T. K. H. Chung, "Women's Attitudes on Human Papillomavirus Vaccination to Their Daughters," *Journal of Adolescent Health* 41 (2007): 204–207.

5. D. S. Cox, A. D. Cox, L. Sturm, and G. Zimet, "Behavioral Interventions to Increase HPV Vaccination Acceptability among Mothers of Young Girls," *Journal of Health Psychology* 29 (2010): 29–39.

6. A genre of radio drama in Spanish.

7. D. Kepka, G. D. Coronado, H. P. Rodriguez, and B. Thompson, "Evaluation of a Radionovela to Promote HPV Vaccine Awareness and Knowledge among Hispanic Parents," *Journal of Community Health* 36 (2011): 957–965.

8. J. R. Cates, A. Shafer, S. J. Diehl, and A. M. Deal, "Evaluating a County-Sponsored Social Marketing Campaign to Increase Mothers' Initiation of HPV Vaccine for Their Pre-Teen Daughters in a Primarily Rural Area," *Social Marketing Quarterly* 17 (2011): 4–26.

9. N. Andersson, A. Cockcroft, N. M. Ansari, K. Omer, M. Baloch, A. Ho Foster, et al. "Evidence-based Discussion Increases Childhood Vaccination Uptake: A Randomised Cluster Controlled Trial of Knowledge Translation in Pakistan," *BMC International Health and Human Rights* 9, suppl. 1 (2009): S8.

10. N. J. Goldstein, R. B. Cialdini, and V. Griskevicius, "A Room with a Viewpoint: Using Social Norms to Motivate Environmental Conservation in Hotels," *Journal of Consumer Research* 35 (2008): 472–482.

11. K. Attwell and M. Freeman, "I Immunise: An Evaluation of a Values-based Campaign to Change Attitudes and Beliefs," *Vaccine* 33 (2015): 6235–6240.

12. J. Schoeppe, A. Cheadle, M. Melton, T. Faubion, C. Miller, J. Matthys, et al., "The Immunity Community: A Community Engagement Strategy for Reducing Vaccine Hesitancy," *Health Promotion Practice* 18 (2017): 654–661.

13. C. Wallace, J. Leask, and L. J. Trevena, "Effects of a Web Based Decision Aid on Parental Attitudes to MMR Vaccination: A Before and After Study," *BMJ* 332 (2006): 146–149.

14. B. Nyhan and J. Reifler, "When Corrections Fail: The Persistence of Political Misperceptions," *Political Behavior* 32 (2010): 303–330.

15. B. Nyhan, J. Reifler, and P. A. Ubel, "The Hazards of Correcting Myths about Health Care Reform," *Medical Care* 51 (2013): 127–132.

16. B. Nyhan, J. Reifler, S. Richey, and G. L. Freed, "Effective Messages in Vaccine Promotion: A Randomized Trial," *Pediatrics* 133 (2014): e835–42.

17. J. Sarlin, "Anti-Vaccination Conspiracy Theories Thrive on Amazon," CNN Business, February 27, 2019, www.cnn.com/2019/02/27/tech/amazon-anti-vaccine-books-movies/index.html.

18. Vaccinate California, http://vaccinatecalifornia.org/.

19. "Senators Richard Pan and Ben Allen to Introduce Legislation to End California's Vaccine Exemption Loophole," February 4, 2015, https://sd26.senate.ca.gov/news/2015-02-04-senators-richard-pan-and-ben-allen-introduce-legislation-end-california-s-vaccine.

20. California Legislative Information, "AB 2109-Pupils: Pupils with a Temporary Disability: Individual Instruction: Pupils Who Are Terminally Ill: Honorary Diplomas," https://leginfo.legislature.ca.gov/faces/billTextClient.xhtml?bill_id=201720180AB2109.

21. California Legislative Information, "SB-277 Public Health: Vaccinations (2015–2016)," https://leginfo.legislature.ca.gov/faces/billCompareClient.xhtml?bill_id=201520160SB277.

22. H. Wiley and S. Bollag, "'Blood Is on Your Hands': Anti-Vaccine Activist Who Tossed Menstrual Cup on Senators Released," *Sacramento Bee*, September 13, 2019, www.sacbee.com/news/politics-government/capitol-alert/article235084637.html.

23. Her personal information was discovered by anti-vaccine activists and placed online.

Chapter 20

1. This is an imperfect method, but it has high accuracy overall. There are, of course, many exceptions where a given name cannot predict gender.

2. N. Smith and T. Graham, "Mapping the Anti-Vaccination Movement on Facebook," *Information, Communication, & Society* (2017) 1–18.

3. Pew Research Center, "83% Say Measles Vaccine Is Safe for Healthy Children," February 9, 2015, www.people-press.org/2015/02/09/83 -percent-say-measles-vaccine-is-safe-for-healthy-children/.

4. There seems to be a misconception that "crunchy" liberals make up the majority of the anti-vaccine movement; however, this is not the case.

5. S. M. Bianchi, L. C. Sayer, M. A. Milkie, and J. P. Robinson, "Housework: Who Did, Does or Will Do It, and How Much Does It Matter?" *Social Forces* 91 (2012): 55–63.

6. US Department of Labor, "General Facts on Women and Job-based Health," 2012.

7. T. S. Tomeny, C. J. Vargo, and S. El-Toukhy, "Geographic and Demographic Correlates of Autism-Related Anti-Vaccine Beliefs on Twitter, 2009–15," *Social Science & Medicine* 191 (2017): 168–175.

8. P. J. Smith, S. Y. Chu, and L. E. Barker, "Children Who Have Received No Vaccines: Who Are They and Where Do They Live?" *Pediatrics* 114 (2004): 187–195.

9. Y. T. Yang, P. L. Delamater, T. F. Leslie, and M. M. Mello, "Sociodemographic Predictors of Vaccination Exemptions on the Basis of Personal Belief in California," *American Journal of Public Health* 106 (2016): 172–177.

10. D. A. Salmon, L. H. Moulton, S. B. Omer, M. P. DeHart, S. Stokley, and N. A. Halsey, "Factors associated with Refusal of Childhood Vaccines among Parents of School-Aged Children: A Case-Control Study," *Archives of Pediatrics and Adolescent Medicine* 159 (2005): 470–476.

Chapter 21

1. J. Haidt and C. Joseph, "Intuitive Ethics: How Innately Prepared Intuitions Generate Culturally Variable Virtues," *Daedalus* 133 (2004): 55–66.

Chapter 22

1. C. Vigeant, "Why I'm Not Afraid to Admit I Used to Be an Anti-Vaxxer," Medium.com, December 11, 2016, https://medium.com/@csaveeg/why -im-not-afraid-to-admit-i-used-to-be-an-anti-vaxxer-3df57b8afcc9.

2. Jane Ridley, "I Was an Anti-Vax Crackpot—until This Happened," *New York Post*, September 20, 2016, https://nypost.com/2016/09/20/i -was-an-anti-vax-crackpot-until-this-happened/.

3. "From Anti-Vax to Pro-Vax: One Mom's Journey," Voices for Vaccines, February 3, 2013, www.voicesforvaccines.org/from-anti-vax-to-pro-vax/.

4. "Letting Go of the Paradigm of Fear," Voices for Vaccines, March 18, 2013, www.voicesforvaccines.org/letting-go-of-the-paradigm-of-fear/.

5. "Leaving the Anti-Vaccine Movement," Voices for Vaccines, February 10, 2014, www.voicesforvaccines.org/leaving-the-anti-vaccine-movement/.

6. "I Was Duped by the Anti-Vaccine Movement," Voices for Vaccines, June 15, 2014, www.voicesforvaccines.org/i-was-duped-by-the-anti-vaccine -movement/.

7. "Manipulated by Fear," Voices for Vaccines, March 7, 2016, https:// www.voicesforvaccines.org/1793-2/.

8. "A Mother I Never Met Changed My Mind about Vaccines," Voices for Vaccines, February 7, 2017, www.voicesforvaccines.org/mother -never-met-changed-mind-vaccines/.

9. "A Horrible Cough and My Vaccination Education," Voices for Vaccines, April 9, 2018, www.voicesforvaccines.org/a-horrible-cough-and -my-vaccination-education/.

Index

About the Author

Jonathan M. Berman, PhD, is an assistant professor at a medical school, where he teaches medical students and does research. In 2017 he was one of the national co-chairs of the March for Science. He lives somewhere with his dog, who shall remain unnamed.